ST. BA RARY

WES '837

SCHOOL OF MEDICINE AND
DENTISTRY LIBRARY
ST. BARTHOLOMEW'S HOSPITAL
WEST SMITHFIELD, EC1A 7BE
This B WEBRENEWAL – www.library.qmul.ac.uk e the
latest ENQUIRIES – 020 7882 8188

Breast Cytopathology

Breast Cytopathology

A diagnostic atlas

Edited by
Peter A. Trott MA, MB BChir, FRCPath
Royal Marsden Hospital and the London Clinic
London
UK

CHAPMAN & HALL MEDICAL
London · Glasgow · Weinheim · New York · Tokyo · Melbourne · Madras

Published by Chapman & Hall, 2–6 Boundary Row, London SE1 8HN, UK

Chapman & Hall, 2–6 Boundary Row, London SE1 8HN, UK

Blackie Academic & Professional, Wester Cleddens Road, Bishopbriggs, Glasgow G64 2NZ, UK

Chapman & Hall GmbH, Pappelallee 3, 69469 Weinheim, Germany

Chapman & Hall USA, 115 Fifth Avenue, New York, NY 10003, USA

Chapman & Hall Japan, ITP-Japan, Kyowa Building, 3F, 2-2-1 Hirakawacho, Chiyoda-ku, Tokyo 102, Japan

Chapman & Hall Australia, 102 Dodds Street, South Melbourne, Victoria 3205, Australia

Chapman & Hall India, R. Seshadri, 32 Second Main Road, CIT East, Madras 600 035, India

First edition 1996

© 1996 Chapman & Hall

Typeset in 10/12pt Palatino by Keyset Composition, Colchester, Essex
Printed in Hong Kong by Dua Hua Printing Press Co., Ltd.

ISBN 0 412 28280 1

Contents

List of contributors   vi

Foreword   vii

Acknowledgements   viii

Preface   ix

1   **Introduction**   1
Peter A. Trott

2   **Benign appearances**   13
Grace McKee

3   **Malignant appearances**   35
Peter A. Trott

4   **Equivocal appearances**   49
Peter A. Trott

5   **Uncommon lesions**   87
Clive A. Wells

6   **Nipple smears**   109
Grace McKee

7   **Efficacy of breast needle aspiration cytodiagnosis**   121
Peter A. Trott

8   **Image-guided fine needle aspiration of impalpable breast lesions**   125
Joan Lamb and Euphemia McGoogan

9   **Research techniques and applications**   137
Ian O. Ellis

Index   153

Contributors

Dr Ian O. Ellis, MB BS, MRCPath,
Department of Histopathology,
City Hospital,
Nottingham, UK

Dr Joan Lamb, MB BCh, DObst RCOG, FRCPath,
Pathology Department,
University of Edinburgh,
Edinburgh, UK

Dr Euphemia McGoogan, MB BCh, FRCPath,
Pathology Department,
University of Edinburgh,
Edinburgh, UK

Dr Grace McKee, MB BS, FRCPath,
Department of Cytopathology,
Royal Surrey County Hospital,
Guildford, UK

Dr Peter A. Trott, MA, MB BChir, FRCPath,
Department of Cytopathology,
The Royal Marsden Hospital,
London, UK

Dr Clive A. Wells, MA, MB BS, MRCPath,
Department of Cytopathology,
St Bartholomew's Hospital,
London, UK

Foreword

As the first chapter of this book illustrates, aspiration cytology of the breast had its tentative beginnings in the middle of the last century, but it was not until eighty years later that a systematic approach to the use of the technique in breast diseases was attempted, with creditable results. However, it was not until the late 1940s, following the seminal publications of Papanicolaou and Traut on the cytologic diagnosis of uterine cancer, that the applicability of cytology to the diagnosis of cancer in general became recognized, culminating in the surge of interest of the last two decades in fine needle aspiration cytology.

Now, lesions in all parts of the body, including those deeply situated in the breast, are amenable to cytological investigation. Today, there can be few persons dealing with breast disease who are unaware of the potential and practicality of diagnosing neoplastic and non-neoplastic lesions of the breast by the methods of cytopathology.

The cytological study of nipple discharge has a similar history: early sporadic reports of cancer cells in nipple discharge, regarded as of academic interest only and hence of little or no practical importance, followed many years later by an outstanding contribution on the subject by Papanicolaou and colleagues. Then a long period of rather low level activity.

Although the literature that has now accumulated on these subjects is substantial, few monographs on the cytopathology of the breast have been published, and even fewer cover the subject in such breadth and detail as this multiauthored work. The authors bring a wealth of experience in histopathology and cytopathology of the breast to this publication. They are seasoned practitioners whose broad background in their discipline has served them well in dealing with the demands and difficulties of cytopathology. Not only are they capable diagnosticians, they are also experienced expositors who have shared widely their knowledge and expertise by the written and the spoken word. Their extensive interest in the cytopathology of the breast is reflected in the scope of this monograph, which includes descriptions of the cytological manifestations of a wide range of conditions, both neoplastic and non-neoplastic. The authors have expressed themselves lucidly, and their text is well supplied with excellent illustrations and generous and appropriate references.

For those who are about to embark on the cytopathology of the breast as well as those who already have experience in the field, this book will serve as an invaluable guide and reference.

Bernard Naylor
Professor of Pathology
University of Michigan
Ann Arbor, Michigan

Acknowledgements

I would like to thank my secretary, Mrs Bridget McCarthy, for her assistance and Mr K. H. Peh for undertaking the literature research. I would also like to acknowledge the cooperation and enthusiasm of many surgeons and physicians for referring specimens for diagnosis, notably Mr Alan McKinna, Dr Trevor Powles, Mr Harvey White and Professor Michael Baum.

Peter Trott

Preface

The aim of this atlas is to illustrate and document an important advance in breast tissue diagnosis that has occurred over the last twenty years. This advance was inspired in Scandinavia, enthusiastically followed on the continent of Europe and finally established in Britain and the USA within the last ten years. The Royal College of Pathologists has embraced fine needle aspiration cytodiagnosis into its training and examination schedules so that nowadays aspiring histopathologists will expect to be examined in this subject and questioned about their experience and ability at interview.

The ability to interpret material aspirated from solid breast lesions ranges from the straightforward to the extremely difficult depending on a multitude of factors which will be addressed in this atlas. The subject has recently been expanded by the acknowledgement that aspiration cytodiagnosis is an important component in the detection of breast cancer through the establishment of the National Health Service Breast Cancer Screening Project. Women presenting for screening often have lumps in the breast that they do not know about and samples from impalpable lesions can now be aspirated safely under image guidance.

This book is designed for those involved in interpreting breast needle aspirates and nipple smears whether they be cytotechnologists or cytopathologists. The atlas describes well-established criteria of diagnosis and has a section on the analysis of those specimens showing equivocal results whereby the authors' experience can be of help to those confronted with difficult problems of interpretation. In addition using this technique has allowed the *in vivo* examination of tissue from solid tumours thereby expanding the possibilities for research using modern investigative techniques.

Peter A. Trott
London, UK
October 1995

1. Introduction

Peter A. Trott

HISTORICAL ASPECTS

The practice of aspiration cytodiagnosis of solid tumours is the modern renaissance of a technique which became eclipsed in 1869, when Klebs [1] invented the method of embedding pieces of tissue in paraffin wax so that thin slices could be cut and stained for histopathological examination. Before then, enterprising investigators had performed 'microscopy' on tissue imprinted or scraped off the cut surface of specimens using the optical instruments of the time. Although Hans and Zacharias Jannsen devised the compound microscope in Middleburg, Holland, in around 1590 [2], the principle appears to have been adapted mostly to building telescopes. The first report of microscopic observations of structures was Micrographia [3], published by Robert Hooke in 1665 that was read and enjoyed by Samuel Pepys. Hooke examined sections of cork and plant stems and even recorded the size of structures with a primitive micrometer. The next landmark is the work and observations of Van Leeuwenhoek [4], who was born in Delft in 1632 and who concentrated on using good quality lenses which he ground himself from quartz. Van Leeuwenhoek was elected Fellow of The Royal Society in 1680 and it is thought that the quality of his instruments was good enough to see protozoa and bacteria.

After this enthusiasm, interest in the subject appears to have waned and it was not until 1826 that Lord Lister's father, Joseph Jackson Lister, a London wine merchant, made great advances when he incorporated sound optical principles into the design of a compound microscope in which chromatic and spherical aberration were largely abolished. He and the Guy's physician, Thomas Hodgkin published a paper [5] on their observations in 1827 and gradually cytodiagnosis was re-introduced into medical practice and in 1836, Johannes Müller published the first valid illustrations of tumour cells [6]. Gradually, through the activities of Schleiden [7] and Schwann [8] and Virchow [9] the concept of 'cellular pathology' evolved.

Needle aspiration cytodiagnosis of the breast

An early advocate of this technique is Skey [10], who in 1850 advocated puncture by a needle of a breast lump which turned out to be a cyst, but evidently no microscopy was undertaken. However, Sir James Paget, in 1853 [11] and Erichsen [12] in the same year, described the microscopic examination of tissue aspirated by a narrow needle from a breast mass. Erichsen, from University College Hospital London reported seven examples of mastectomy performed for chronic abscess diagnosed by needle aspiration which simulated a scirrhous carcinoma. Paget, in his *Lectures on Tumours* [13] eloquently describes the appearances of single cancer cells under the microscope. Augustine Prichard, a Bristol surgeon, used a grooved needle to assess breast lumps and describes the cytology of fat necrosis in a book published in 1863 [14].

After the birth of histology, the old cytological methods lingered on, despite the increased amount of information that could be obtained from examining histopathological specimens. In the 1920s, Dudgeon and Patrick at St Thomas' Hospital [15] developed the 'wet film' technique whereby the cells from the freshly cut surface of an excised surgical specimen were fixed in Schaudinn's solution and stained in Mayer's haemalum and eosin for microscopic examination and diagnosis. This was thought to be as accurate as frozen section in the examination of breast specimens. At the same time at the Memorial Hospital in New York, Martin and Ellis [16] investigated the usefulness and accuracy of needle aspiration cytodiagnosis of a large number of subcutaneous masses including the breast. Breast needle cytodiagnosis continues at this hospital where it was embraced by the pathologists Ewing and Stewart who correlated the appearances of the aspirated cells with the counterpart histopathology and enumerated guidelines for its practice [17].

Since 1950, research and clinical correlation of the technique of aspiration cytodiagnosis have occurred in Stockholm at the Radiumhemmet department of the Karolinska hospital [18]. Here, largely as a result of the recognition of its worth by radiotherapists, and the vision and enthusiasm of Josef Zajicek (Fig. 1.1) the place for a rapid method of preoperative diagnosis was appreciated and developed, despite initial scepticism by pathologists. At this hospital and other centres in Scandinavia, there are now departments of 'Clinical Cytology' to which patients with breast lumps and other subcutaneous nodules are referred for cytodiagnosis. The cytopathologist palpates the nodule and then aspirates it thereby ensuring that a good quality sample is obtained. In 1968, Franzen and Zajicek [19] reported a review of 3479 breast aspirates examined in this way. In the United Kingdom the advantages of such a clinic are being appreciated and this arrangement is working very successfully at district hospitals as well as specialist centres. There are also reports of cytopathologists in the United States establishing cyto-

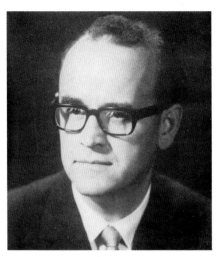

Figure 1.1 Josef Zajicek, Cytopathologist, Karolynska Institute, Stockholm, 1923–1979.
(*by permission Acta Cytologica, Williams & Wilkins*)

logy clinics to which clinicians refer patients for cytodiagnosis [20].

The recognition of the special training and expertise required in cytodiagnosis is reflected by the establishment in 1989 of a Special Certificate of Cytology in the USA, and the introduction by the Royal College of Pathologists in the United Kingdom of a Diploma in Cytopathology in 1993.

THE PLACE OF ASPIRATION CYTODIAGNOSIS IN THE MANAGEMENT OF BREAST DISEASE

It is the purpose of breast fine needle aspiration cytodiagnosis to identify patients having malignant disease with a positive predictive value of 100 per cent and to provide a diagnostic sensitivity of similar accuracy, in conjunction with clinical examination and mammography. The test is comparatively painless for the patient and enables a result to be available at best within a few minutes. Although a recent review of the specificity and sensitivity of results reported in the literature by Giard [21] showed a wide range of diagnostic accuracy, many papers have shown a positive predictive value for the diagnosis of carcinoma of 100 per cent with a range of sensitivity between 65 and 98 per cent (see Chapter 7).

The difficulty for the clinician examining the breast is to distinguish between a patient with diffuse nodularity and a discrete mass. A palpable mass can be easily aspirated, especially one that is tethered to the skin or underlying tissue, whereas nodular lesions without a dominant mass leaves the clinician uncertain where to insert the needle. Although multiple aspirates may resolve this problem, radiological imaging can help in this predicament both with regard to mammography, in which a dominant lesion can be identified and subsequently palpated and to ultrasonography which can be undertaken in conjunction with needle aspiration cytodiagnosis on the outpatient couch. The latter technique, which is gaining popularity, has the advantage that the position of the needle in the breast can be seen during the procedure and thus its direction controlled. Unfortunately, microcalcification which is so important for the identification of breast cancers, cannot be seen at ultrasound imaging.

The aspiration of fluid from a cyst, thought by all to be a carcinoma, will bring an expression of joy to the face of the patient and a sense of relief to the clinician. The patient can be both reassured and cured of the breast lump. A review of a large number of cases of breast cyst aspiration cytodiagnosis by Ciatto [22] indicated that the routine cytological examination of breast fluid aspirated from all cysts is unnecessary and certainly not cost effective. These authors reviewed 6782 cyst fluids from 4105 patients in which five clinically and radiologically inapparent intracystic papillomas were detected all of which produced blood-stained fluid, although the cytology was negative in two of these cases. Although one incidental case of occult lobular carcinoma *in situ* was detected in this review, all the cancers identified had been suspected by physical examination and or mammography. Reports support classical teaching [23] that fluid aspirated from a breast cyst should be examined cytologically when it is discoloured, particularly blood stained and when the lump persists after aspiration. Medullary carcinoma frequently produces blood-stained fluid when needled.

There are many studies that have demonstrated that the combination of breast aspiration, mammography and clinical examination detects almost all cancers [24]. In addition, this 'triple approach' [25, 26] reduces the number of frozen sections requested to the histopathology department, and of course provides a preoperative diagnosis of malignancy so that treatment can be discussed with the patient before the operation and consent for treatment obtained. Layfield in an editorial in the *American Journal of Clinical Pathology* [27] concurs with this 'triple diagnosis' technique and recommends, in addition, physical re-examination between three and six months later.

Strong links between cytopathologist and clinician are essential and in most centres this is manifested in encouragement to complete request forms fully and legibly and include the clinical diagnosis and to present cases at clinicopathological meetings. At Nottingham [28], this is taken one stage further and breast aspirates are categorized by clinicians as 'A', 'B', or 'C'. 'A' category indicates a clinical diagnosis of carcinoma, 'B' of benign changes and 'C' is a safety category to include such specific entities as fibroadenoma or abscess. All request forms require this categorization and in this way clinicians are constrained to diagnose and cytopathologists can construct a report. It is a maxim however, that cytopathological specimens (and histopathological sections for that matter) should be examined microscopically **before** reading the request form, but never reported **without knowing** the clinical details. In this way the significance of the observations of the microscopist will not tend to be overruled by knowledge of the clinical diagnosis and the ultimate report will be appropriate.

The complications of aspiration cytodiagnosis include local haematoma, which can be largely prevented by firm pressure for about two minutes after withdrawing the needle, and pneumothorax, which was reported in a review [29] to have occurred in seven patients with an incidence of four per hundred aspirates. Not all clinicians claim to have seen this high a rate of pneumothorax and indeed in a recent review of 48 Italian Institutions [30] involving over 200 000 needle aspirates an incidence of 0.01 per cent was reported. It must be admitted however, that many such punctures will go undetected.

Tumour seeding along the needle tract is of mainly theoretical interest as most carcinomas will be at least excised or given other forms of treatment. Suffice to say that in this latter group no seeding has been reported and indeed there is experimental evidence from Eriksson et al. [31] who aspirated tumours in mice that seeding may only occur under extreme test conditions and that there was no increase in the death rate from increased tumour dissemination.

In the diagnosis of breast disease, aspiration cytodiagnosis must be compared with needle biopsy whereby a core of tissue is obtained for histopathological examination [32]. The advantages of this latter technique are that infiltrative carcinoma and other histological sub-types can be identified, and to a limited degree, that the grade of carcinoma can be assessed. To a tissue pathologist trained in histo-pathology this kind of tissue is more familiar than a needle aspirate. However, rapid progress is being made in the United Kingdom in the training of histopathologists in the interpretation of cells obtained by fine needle aspiration. Although the Biopty-gun is less painful than the Tru-cut needle biopsy which uses a 14-gauge needle, the sensitivity is far lower than that obtained with the Tru-cut needle and probably not that much better than a fine needle aspirate. However, when a needle aspirate has failed in a suspected carcinoma it is wise to proceed to a Biopty-gun biopsy although this procedure is very difficult in tumours less than 1.5 cm in diameter.

The relative advantages of breast aspiration cytodiagnosis and histopathological diagnosis by core biopsy was the subject of an editorial by Howell [33] who highlights the advantages of breast cytodiagnosis even in patients having conservation therapy. She emphasizes that proper interpretation through education is required in an efficient breast aspiration cytodiagnosis service, which is safe, comparatively painless and cost effective.

There are two groups of patients in whom breast aspiration cytodiagnosis of solid breast nodules is particularly important and often overlooked. In younger patients aged under 35 years, mammography is often unsatisfactory because of the denseness of the breast and not recommended due to the risk of radiation exposure. In addition, the clinician is often inclined to discount a diagnosis of cancer, as this is an uncommon diagnosis. The commonest cause of a lump in the breast in a young person is a fibroadenoma which can be conclusively diagnosed by aspiration cytodiagnosis, as of course can carcinoma which may be quite unexpected. In a review [34] of 150 women aged less than 35 years, aspiration cytodiagnosis was the best method for diagnosing carcinoma compared with clinical and mammographic diagnosis. In another review [35] of aspirates of breast lesions in women aged 30 and under, the presence of epithelial atypia revealed four carcinomas identified at histopathological biopsy, and in three other patients a definitive diagnosis of carcinoma was made by aspiration cytodiagnosis.

The second group of patients where aspiration cytodiagnosis should not be overlooked is in elderly patients in whom the diagnosis of cancer by this method can be the only invasive procedure necessary. Some patients are conveniently treated only by endocrine therapy, which may control tumour growth sufficiently to ensure good quality of life.

ASSOCIATION WITH HISTOPATHOLOGY

Although cytopathologists involved in breast fine needle aspiration cytodiagnosis are less concerned with histopathological classifications than with the diagnosis of malignancy, a thorough understanding of the histopathological appearances of breast disease is essential for correct cytological interpretation. This is because individual epithelial cells in quite benign lesions can have alarming appearances and it is easy to imagine how a misdiagnosis of malignancy might be made when such cells are aspirated.

The histopathological diagnosis of ductal hyperplasia, particularly of the atypical variant is made when either the cytological or pattern criteria of ductal carcinoma *in situ* are met but both are not 'present in full flower' to quote from Page and Anderson's authoritative book [36] on this subject. Consequently aspirates from these benign lesions may contain large pleomorphic irregular cells indistinguishable from those seen in cases of ductal carcinoma *in situ*. The pattern component of swirling and streaming, characteristic of ductal hyperplasia will not be appreciated in aspirate specimens.

However, within the smear, provided it is a good quality specimen, there will be unequivocal benign cells both ductal epithelial and myoepithelial, many of the latter appearing as pairs of bare nuclei. For this reason the diagnostic cytopathologist must be circumspect when only a few groups of highly atypical cells are present and a suspicious report issued.

Moreover, Stanley *et al.* [37] have found no correlation between proliferative atypical lesions seen on histological examination with appearances in needle aspirates; in other words, there is so far no evidence that equivocal appearances in smears correlates with precancerous lesions subsequently identified histologically.

The epithelium lining the clefts in fibroadenomas appears hyperplastic and shows mitotic activity not uncommonly. Aspirates from these lesions may show very atypical appearances and some have been misdiagnosed as carcinoma [38]. The histopathologist has the advantage of seeing the complete pattern of the lesion whether it is pericanalicular or intracanalicular and so making the diagnosis, whereas in aspirates such features are not evident. However, when three components are identified in aspirates consisting of epithelial cells in a 'stag's horn' pattern, stroma that stains metachromatically with May–Grünwald Giemsa and numerous myoepithelial cells, many singly and in pairs, the appearances will be diagnostic of fibroadenoma (see Chapter 2).

In patients having recent radiotherapy there may be much individual cellular atypia that has been well described histologically [39]. As well as showing evidence of proliferation, individual cells may be very large and have macronucleoli. In these cases knowledge of the clinical history is essential and can avoid a false positive diagnosis. A knowledge of the histological appearances of cells lining benign breast cysts which can be squamous or apocrine metaplastic, will also help in interpreting the abnormalities often seen in cell clusters aspirated from cysts.

Although there are a large number of case reports of the cytological appearances of tissue aspirated from rare and unusual benign and malignant tumours, there has been little prospective correlation between the cytological appearances of cells in breast aspirates and the subsequent histopathology. However, certain types of tumour do have characteristic cytological appearances, the best example of which is colloid or mucinous adenocarcinoma. In the smears from these lesions the mucus stains bright purple in May–Grünwald Giemsa and so provides the clue to the diagnosis. Very often the carcinoma cells are small and comparatively insignificant although with experience it will be noted that only one type of cell is present and some nuclei do indeed show atypia. Cytopathologists can be confident in predicting the histology in which the typical features are seen although of course the colloid component may be focal rather than the 90 per cent of the tumour volume required to make the diagnosis of a tumour associated with a comparatively good prognosis.

Medullary carcinoma with lymphoid stroma will also have characteristic features in an aspirate in which plasma cells are identified as well as large pleomorphic poorly differentiated carcinoma cells with prominent nucleoli. The prospective correlation with histopathology in these cases is less certain. In another example, cytopathologists will often find that cases showing clumps of small closely packed but irregular cells in the aspirate that are difficult to interpret turn out to be infiltrating lobular carcinoma. Although there are some characteristic features, a prospective histopathological diagnosis is only sometimes possible and the cytologist will be more concerned to establish a diagnosis of malignancy rather than its histopathological type.

The problem of the influence of cancer histology on the success of fine needle aspiration cytodiagnosis has been investigated by Lamb and Anderson [40]. They found in an analysis of 1318 infiltrating not otherwise specified (NOS) carcinomas that carcinoma was identified in 84 per cent of cases.

Although mucoid and medullary cancers were diagnosed only slightly less often, in tubular, cribriform, lobular and non-invasive ductal cancer, malignancy was only recognized in 60–70 per cent of cases.

A thorough knowledge of breast histopathology will also teach the novice cytologist the variety of patterns and cell types seen in breast carcinoma. Thus, the presence of elongated spindly sarcoma-like cells will not always be from a stromal lesion, but will reflect the metaplastic potential of malignant breast epithelium and be a component of carcinoma. Similarly osteoclast-like giant cells are seen quite often [41] which have shown to be KP1 (CD68) positive [42] providing support for the histiocytic origin of these cells.

TECHNIQUES

Who does it and where should it be done?

There is controversy over whether it is best that the clinician (surgeon or physician) performs breast needle aspiration or the pathologist who will also undertake the microscopic interpretation [43–45]. For years surgeons have been aspirating breast cysts in clinics; the procedure is diagnostic and often curative. It is also true that the consistency of the tumour can be revealed by fine needle aspiration and lumps that are rubbery and 'grip' the needle and so prevent its being withdrawn easily are more often benign and come from fibrotic fibrocystic change. On the other hand carcinomas will feel 'gritty' so that the operator achieves an additional physical sign which enhances the clinical diagnosis.

The pathologist is also concerned with physical signs and indeed whoever aspirates a lump also palpates it and therefore has the opportunity to make a clinical diagnosis. Furthermore, like clinicians, the pathologist can talk to the patient and thereby take a history of the condition according to classical time-honoured medical procedures. However, the pathologist is more knowledgeable about the type of preparation that is required on the slide in order to achieve perfect staining whether it be Papanicolaou staining (equivalent to haematoxylin and eosin) or Giemsa, which is the classic stain of the haematology department. In order to achieve satisfactory staining the smear must be prepared correctly as each method has totally contrasting preparatory procedures.

In order to achieve perfect Papanicolaou-stained smears the material has to be fixed before it dries, using the usual gynaecological spray-fix, whereas smears destined to be stained with Giemsa must dry instantaneously and in some laboratories a hair dryer is provided for this purpose. The consequence of this is that smears destined for Papanicolaou staining that dry before they are fixed give poor results and smears destined for Giemsa that do not dry quickly also provide poor results.

In practice, smears earmarked for Papanicolaou staining should be smeared on the slide rather thicker than those destined for Giemsa staining, and consequently the pathologist who is knowledgeable about the techniques may be the best person to perform the needle aspirate.

In Scandinavia under a scheme pioneered at the Karolinska Hospital, all patients requiring needle aspiration cytology including those of the breast, are referred to the Cytology Clinic. This practice is the most important reason for the high quality of the aspiration cytology service throughout Scandinavia that consistently achieves very high levels of specificity and sensitivity.

The Cytology Clinic is an autonomous unit staffed by nurses and secretaries as well as pathologists to whom the patient is referred. Not only hospital clinicians but also general practitioners have access to these clinics and the reports are referred back appropriately. The pathologist can make use of his clinical training and may not only take a full history and even look at X-rays, but palpate the mass and perform appropriate investigations such as transillumination or even auscultation if it is thought to be necessary. In this way the pathologist has the best of both worlds. He has made a clinical diagnosis, and has obtained the specimen that is required before he does the microscopy.

In the United Kingdom pathologists are appreciating the advantages of this arrangement which has been welcomed by clinicians. The costs of the tests have been shown to be much reduced not only because unsatisfactory specimens are extremely rare, but also because more definitive diagnoses can be achieved. Notable examples of this procedure are at Northampton in Dr Coghill's Laboratory [46], The University College Hospital in London in Dr Kocjan's Laboratory [47] and several other centres.

In the United States similar clinics are also being established. One is in San Francisco which is designed along Scandinavian guidelines and has reported excellent results [20]. Over a seven-year period there has been a twenty-fold increase in the number of patients submitted to this clinic for examination. Specimens consist mainly of breast aspirates but include thyroid, soft tissue subcutaneous lumps, salivary gland tumours and prostate.

Surgeons are reluctant to lose the extra physical signs that they obtain from aspirating tumours themselves and a compromise solution is where the pathologist attends the surgical clinic in order that the best, properly prepared specimens are obtained [48]. This has the advantage of speed and thereby convenience for the patient who will discover during the clinic and after consultation with the surgeon what her management will be. This 'immediate reporting' technique does not require such a radical reorganization as the establishment of an autonomous clinic and it is therefore the established method in several centres in the United Kingdom.

How is it done?

It is the purpose of aspiration cytodiagnosis to transfer cells from the lesion onto a slide in such a way that they can be stained and diagnosed. In achieving this many methods are available ranging from the use of a syringe holder to simply inserting a hypodermic needle into a lesion and subsequently squirting the material that has been collected in its bore onto a slide [49]. The syringe holder has been used widely in Scandinavia, and there are other devices available, mostly designed by surgeons, to enable them to aspirate conveniently.

The syringe holder (Fig. 1.2) requires a certain dexterity to use it properly, but once this has been mastered it is a useful device that increases the yield and presumably the accuracy of the technique. However, many practitioners consider that simply using a 10 ml syringe with a green (20-gauge) or blue (22-gauge) hypodermic needle is equally suitable (Fig. 1.3).

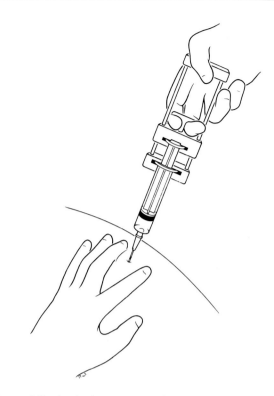

Figure 1.2 Aspirating a mass using a syringe holder.

Figure 1.3 Aspirating a mass using a 10 ml syringe. Note that a small volume of air has been sucked into the syringe before the mass is aspirated.

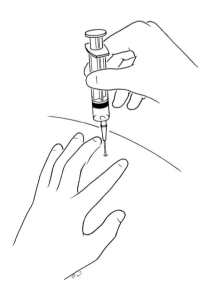

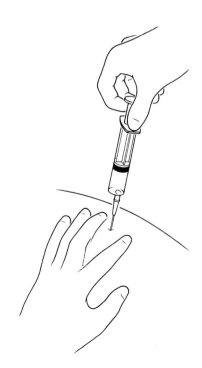

The recommended method is as follows:

1. Clean the skin and fix the breast lump between finger and thumb or between fingers with the patient preferably supine.
2. Draw up about 2 ml of air into the syringe and ensure that the needle is firmly fixed into the barrel of the syringe to avoid an air leakage.
3. Insert the needle tip into the centre of the lesion.
4. Aspirate with a lot of negative pressure in the syringe, up to 9 or even 10 ml, while moving the needle tip within the tumour which should be kept fixed between finger and thumb or fingers. This is the critical part of the operation. Some large tumours may be necrotic in their centres so it is wise to aspirate round the periphery if this can be identified. It is also important to aspirate in many directions so that samples from different areas of the tumour are aspirated (Fig. 1.4). Such wide sampling is not possible when performing a needle biopsy for histopathological diagnosis, and it may well be that a larger volume of tissue is obtained through the fine needle aspiration technique.
6. It is extremely important to release the negative pressure in the syringe before extracting the needle from the tumour. If this is not done, then, as the needle is pulled through the skin, air will rush in and the contents of the needle will be blown into the barrel of the syringe and will be difficult to extract.
7. Make blobs at the ends of several slides and smear appropriately remembering that those des-

tined for Papanicolaou staining should be rather thick and those for Giemsa staining thin.
8. The syringe contents and needle contents are now rinsed into buffered saline or culture medium for centrifugating for special stains or research purposes.

The procedure should be undertaken in a confident manner in order to reassure the patient, with a good light and an assistant nearby. From the patient's point of view a slick operation inspires the trust that is born out of the knowledge that the aspirator knows what he is doing.

With regard to the methods of staining no attempt will be made here to set out methods that are adequately covered in standard cytology text books. Particularly recommended are Proctor's chapters in *Clinical Cytotechnology* edited by D. V. Coleman and P. A. Chapman [50], to which the reader is referred. The Papanicolaou technique and the May–Grünwald Giemsa technique are the two standard reference stains for breast samples including cysts, smears and nipple discharge specimens. Centrifugation using the Cytospin is extremely useful for obtaining additional slides for special stains including immunocytochemistry. Furthermore, slides prepared in this way can be stored at −80° centigrade for subsequent staining. This method has been used for samples from patients on primary medical therapy taken sequentially in order to assess biological parameters that may relate to appropriate treatment and prognosis.

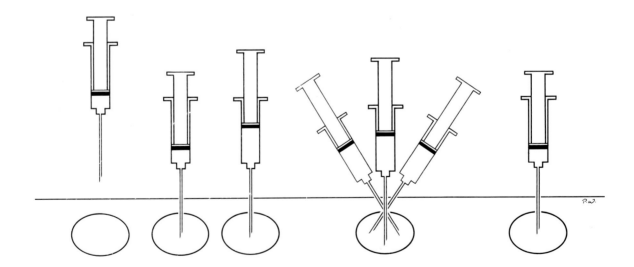

Figure 1.4 Diagrammatic view of the aspiration of a mass in many directions.

REPORTING RESULTS

Breast cytopathology reports should be concise [51] and unambiguous and composed in three sections. The first describes the anatomical site of the specimen, the second (labelled microscopy) describes the microscopic appearances and the third section is the conclusion. This should be a single word and must be a cytopathological diagnosis. Any temptation to make a histopathological diagnosis should be avoided, although it is appropriate to consider this in the descriptive section. Indeed, a diagnosis such as 'malignant lymphoma', unless totally clear-cut from the cytopathological point of view should be considered in the section describing the microscopical appearances, and the lesion concluded to be 'malignant neoplasm'. Similarly, an aspirate showing numerous large spindle and bizarre-shaped cells might be considered to be sarcoma, but spindle cell carcinomas would produce a similar pattern and in the absence of immunocytochemical support for a mesenchymal origin of a tumour its possibility should be discussed in the microscopic section; however, the conclusion again should be 'malignant neoplasm'. This need not be so in other anatomical sites, e.g. the retroperitoneum, but in the breast the possibility of pseudosarcomatous areas or sarcomatous metaplasia within a carcinoma is a well-known phenomenon [52].

When reporting benign disease it is best to conclude 'no evidence of malignancy'. The temptation to provide a diagnosis of 'fibrocystic change' or synonym should be avoided although the description of the cells might lead the clinician to conclude such a diagnosis in consultation with the clinical and mammographic appearances. Despite the appearances of fibroadenoma in needle aspirates being well described and tested prospectively [53], the features should also be described in the microscopic description section and the report concluded 'no evidence of malignancy'. A note will be appropriate, however, in the description to the effect that the appearances are compatible with a fibroadenoma. It is certainly important to identify these lesions as it may not be desirable to excise them for fear of disfiguring the breast, and in consultation with the patient, a surgeon might adopt a policy of observation. Indeed, these lesions can disappear in middle life.

The macroscopic description of the specimen is also important and the aspirator should inform the cytopathologist of the nature of the sample. The presence of fluid in the syringe indicates a cyst, although the deposit may be acellular. An appropriate report in this situation would read, 'Six millilitres of clear fluid aspirated. Microscopy; No cells present. No evidence of malignancy'. When the aspirator is the pathologist such potential difficulties are eliminated but if specimens are sent to the laboratory by surgeons, without clinical information, the report of 'no cells present' indicating an inadequate specimen, would be an incorrect one.

Although it is the aim to provide a definitive diagnosis of malignancy or benignity, this is not always possible although the proportion of equivocal reports will be reduced with experience. Many pathologists have adopted a numerical classification prefixed with the letter 'C' whereby C1 means inadequate, C2 means benign and C5 means malignant. C3 denotes a degree of atypia but is probably benign and C4 is suspicious of malignancy. Detailed definitions of these categories are listed in the National Health Service Breast Screening Programme Manual on 'Guidelines for Cytology Procedures and Reporting in Breast Cancer Screening' [54]. These are reproduced here, with some adaptations.

C1 Inadequate

C1 indicates a scanty or acellular specimen or poor preparation. Scanty cellularity is defined as less than five clumps of epithelial cells, and preparative artefact such as crushing or excessive blood may also be reasons for rejecting a specimen as inadequate. Preparative artefact also includes drying that occurs if smears for Giemsa staining dry too slowly as they are too thick, or when wet fixed smears are allowed to dry before fixation.

C2 Benign

C2 indicates an adequate sample showing no evidence of malignancy and thus if representative warrants a negative report. The specimen should be cellular, i.e. at least five clumps of epithelial cells and they should have the morphological characteristics of benignity. The likelihood of a specific condition should be mentioned, for example fibroadenoma, fat necrosis, granulomatous mastitis or lymph node if sufficient features are present.

C3 Atypia, probably benign

A C3 specimen will have all the characteristics of a benign aspirate with additional features not commonly seen in benign specimens. These would include nuclear pleomorphism, some loss of cohesiveness and nuclear and cytoplasmic changes perhaps resulting from hormonal or treatment influences. The use of this category is arbitrary and the number of cases included reduces with experience.

C4 Suspicious of malignancy

Cases in the C4 group are almost certainly malignant and although the cells are very abnormal, the pathologist feels unable to provide a categorical diagnosis of malignancy. These reservations fall into three main categories. The specimen may be scanty, or poorly preserved, or poorly prepared. Secondly, the sample may show some malignant features but not enough to be considered to make a clear-cut diagnosis. Thirdly, the overall pattern may be benign with large numbers of characteristic duct epithelial and myoepithelial cells, singly and in pairs, but an occasional cluster will be composed of large irregular cells with definite malignant features.

C5 Malignant

C5 indicates malignancy, characteristic of carcinoma or other malignant tumour. The pathologist should 'feel at ease' in making such a diagnosis. Malignancy should not be diagnosed on the basis of a single criterion, but a combination of such features will be necessary to achieve this diagnosis such as those listed in Table 3.1.

REFERENCES

1. Klebs (1869) Die Einschmelzungsmethode, ein Beitrag zur mikroskopischen Technik. *Arch. Mikrosk. Anat. Entw. Mech.* **5**, 164.
2. Bradbury, S. (1967) *The Evolution of the Microscope*, Pergamon, Oxford.
3. Hooke, R. (1665) *Micrographia*.
4. Van der Star, P. (1953) Descriptive catalogue of the simple microscopes in the Riksmuseum voor de Gescheidenis der Natuurwetens Schappen, Leiden.
5. Hodgkin, T. and Lister, J. J. (1827) Notice on some microscopical observations of the blood of animal tissue. *Phil. Mag.* **2**, 130.
6. Müller, J. (1836) Ueber den feineren bau und die Formen der Krankhaften Geschwultzte, Riemer.
7. Schleiden, M. J. (1847) Contributions to phytogenesis. Tr. Smith H. Sydenham Society.
8. Schwann, T. (1847) Microscopical research into the accordance in the structure and growth of animals and plants. Tr. Smith, H. Sydenham Society.
9. Virchow, R. (1860) *Cellular Pathology*. Tr. Chance, F. 2nd edn, Churchill.
10. Skey, F. C. (1850) *Operative Surgery*, Churchill.
11. Paget, J. (1853) *Lectures on Surgical Pathology*, Vol. 2, Longman.
12. Erichsen, J. E. (1853) *The Science and Art of Surgery*, 1st Edn, Walton and Maberly.
13. Paget, J. (1853) *Lectures on Tumours*, Longman.
14. Prichard, A. (1863) Ten years of operative surgery in the provinces, 1850–1860, 875 operations. Part 2, Richards.
15. Dudgeon, L. S. and Patrick, C. V. (1927) A new method for the rapid microscopical diagnosis of tumours. *Br. J. Surg.* **15**, 250.
16. Martin, H. E. and Ellis, E. B. (1930) Biopsy by needle puncture and aspiration. *Ann. Surg.* **92**, 169–81.
17. Stewart, F. W. (1933) The diagnosis of tumours by aspiration. *Am. J. Pathol.* **9**, 801–6.
18. Zajicek, J. (1974) Aspiration biopsy cytology, Part 1. Cytology of supradiaphragmatic organs, in *Monographs in Clinical Cytology* (ed. G. L. Weid), S. Karger, Basel.
19. Franzen, S. L. and Zajicek, J. (1968) Aspiration biopsy in diagnosis of palpable lesions of the breast. Critical review of 3479 consecutive biopsies. *Acta Radiol.* **7**, 241–62.
20. Abele, J. S. and Miller, T. R. (1993) Implementation of an outpatient needle aspiration biopsy service and clinic, in *Cytopathology Annual*, (ed. Waldemar, A. Schmit), Williams and Williams, Baltimore, pp. 43–71.
21. Giard, R. W. M. and Herman, J. O. (1992) The value of aspiration cytologic examination of the breast: a statistical review of the medical literature. *Cancer*, **69**, 2104–10.
22. Ciatto, S., Cariaggi, P. and Bulgaresi, P. (1987) The value of routine cytologic examination of breast cyst fluids. *Acta Cytol.* **31**, 301–4.
23. Haggensen, C. D. (1971) *Diseases of the Breast*, 2nd edn, Saunders Co. Philadelphia p. 172.
24. Thomas, J. M., Fitzharris, B. M., Redding, W. H. *et al.* (1978) Clinical examination, xeromammography and fine needle aspiration cytology in diagnosis of breast lesions. *Br. Med. J.* **2**, 1139–41.
25. Di Pietro, S., Fariselli, G., Bandieramonte, G. *et al.* (1987) Diagnostic efficacy of the clinical-radiological-cytological triplet in solid breast lumps: Results of a second prospective study on 631 patients. *Eur. J. Surg. Oncol.* **13**, 335–50.
26. Dixon, J. M., Anderson, T. J., Lamb, J. *et al.* (1984) Fine needle aspiration cytology in relationship to clinical examination and mammography in the diagnosis of a solid breast mass. *Br. J. Surg.* **71**, 593.
27. Layfield, L. J. H. (1992) Can fine-needle aspiration replace open biopsy in the diagnosis of palpable breast lesions? *Am. J. Clin. Path.* **98**, 145–7.
28. Ellis, I. O., Galea, M. H., Locker, A. *et al.* (1993) Early experience in breast cancer screening: emphasis on development of protocols for triple assessment. *Breast* **2**, 148–53.
29. Gateley, C. A., Maddox, P. R. and Mansel, R. E.

(1991) Pneumothorax: A complication of fine needle aspiration of the breast. *Br. Med. J.* **30**, 627–8.

30. Catania, S., Veronesi, P., Marassi, A. *et al.* (1993) Risk of pneumothorax after fine needle aspiration of the breast: Italian experience of more than 200,000 aspirations. *Breast* **2**, 246–7.

31. Eriksson, O., Hagmar, B. and Ryd, W. (1984) Effects of fine-needle aspiration and other biopsy procedures on tumor dissemination in mice. *Cancer*, **54**, 73–8.

32. Millis, R. R. (1984) Needle biopsy of the breast, in *The Breast*, IAP Monograph No. 25 (eds R. W. McDivitt, H. A. Oberman, L. Ozzello and N. Kaufman) Williams and Wilkins, Baltimore/London, pp. 186–203.

33. Howell, L. P. (1993) Diagnosis of palpable breast cancer by FNA: A changing role? *Diag. Cytopathol.* **9**, 611–2.

34. Yelland, A., Graham, M. D., Trott, P. A. *et al.* (1991) Diagnosing breast carcinoma in young women. *Br. Med. J.* **302**, 618–20.

35. Maygarden, S. J., McCall, J. B. and Frable, W. J. (1991) Fine needle aspiration of breast lesions in women aged 30 and under. *Acta Cytol.* **35**, 687–94.

36. Page, D. L. and Anderson, T. J. (1987) *Diagnostic Histopathology of the Breast*. Churchill Livingstone, Edinburgh, p. 137.

37. Stanley, M. W., Henry-Stanley, M. J. and Zera, R. (1993) Atypia in breast fine needle aspiration smears correlates poorly with the presence of a prognostically significant proliferative lesion of ductal epithelium. *Human Pathol.* **24**, 630–5.

38. Jatoi, I. and Trott, P. A. (1994) False positive reporting in breast fine needle aspiration cytology: incidence and causes. *Breast*, in press.

39. Girling, A. C., Hanby, A. M. and Millis, R. R. (1990) Radiation and other pathological changes in breast tissue after conservation treatment for carcinoma. *J. Clin. Pathol.* **43**, 152–6.

40. Lamb, J. L. and Anderson, T. J. (1989) Influence of cancer histology on the success of FNA of breast. *J. Clin. Pathol.* **42**, 733–9.

41. Dey, P. and Karmarkar, T. (1993) Aspiration cytology of breast carcinoma with multinucleated osteoclast-like giant cells. *Cytopathology* **4**, 382–3.

42. Stewart, C. J. R. and Mutch, A. F. (1991) Breast carcinoma with osteoclast-like giant cells. *Cytopathology*, **2**, 215–9.

43. Stanley, M. W. (1990) Who should perform fine needle aspiration biopsies? *Diagn. Cytopathol.* **6**, 215–7.

44. Lee, K. R., Foster, R. S. and Papillo, J. L. (1987) Cytodiagnosis of classic lobular carcinoma and its variants. *Acta Cytol.* **31**, 281–4.

45. Winship, T. D. (1969) Aspiration biopsy of breast cancers by the pathologist. *Am. J. Clin. Pathol.* **52**, 438–40.

46. Brown, L. A. and Coghill, S. B. (1992) Cost effectiveness of a fine needle aspirate clinic. *Cytopathology*, **3**, 275–80.

47. Kocjan, G. (1991) Evaluation of the cost effectiveness of establishing a fine needle aspiration cytology clinic in a hospital out patient department. *Cytopathology*, **2**, 13–8.

48. Duguid, H. L., Wood, R. A. and Irving, A. D. *et al.* (1979) Needle aspiration of the breast with immediate reporting of material. *Br. Med. J.* **2**, 185–7.

49. Rajasekhar, A., Sundaram, C., Chowdhary, T., *et al.* (1991) Diagnostic utility of fine needle sampling without aspiration: A prospective study. *Diagn. Cytopathol.* **7**, 473–6.

50. Proctor, D. T. (1989) in *Clinical Cytotechnology*, (ed. D. V. Coleman and P. A. Chapman), Butterworths, London, pp. 52–105.

51. Kline, T. S. (1990) Communication and aspiration biopsy cytology: Clear, concise, and to the point. (editorial). *Diagn. Cytopathol.* **6**, 153.

52. Sloane, J. P. (1985) *Biopsy Pathology of the Breast*, Chapman and Hall, London, p. 179.

53. Bottles, K., Chan, J. S., Holly, E. A. *et al.* (1988) Cytologic criteria for fibroadenoma. *Am. J. Clin. Pathol.* **89**, 707–13.

54. Cytology subgroup of the National Coordinating Committee for Breast Cancer Screening Pathology, (eds. C. A. Wells, I. O. Ellis, H. D. Zakhour and A. R. Wilson) (1994) Guidelines for cytology procedures and reporting on fine needle aspirates of the breast. *Cytopathology* **5**, 316–34.

2. Benign appearances

Grace McKee

INTRODUCTION

The breast is an organ which is under the control of hormonal influences. Marked changes occur in the breast at puberty, pregnancy and lactation and after the menopause. The breast starts to develop at the onset of puberty with an increase in both the epithelial component and the fibrofatty stroma. In the premenopausal, non-pregnant woman the breast is composed of a series of branching ducts which collect centrally to form a group of fifteen to twenty larger ducts which open onto the nipple. These larger lactiferous ducts dilate just beneath the nipple to form the lactiferous sinuses which then narrow before opening (Fig. 2.1).

The terminal duct lobular unit comprises a lobule, consisting of a number of acini and its terminal duct and is continuous with segmental ducts that unite to form larger ducts. The acini or lobules are lined by small cuboidal epithelial cells surrounded by a discontinuous layer of myoepithelial cells (Fig. 2.2). The ducts are lined by a layer of slightly larger cuboidal epithelial cells also resting on a layer of myoepithelial cells (Fig. 2.3). This shows the importance of searching for myoepithelial cells in cytological preparations as a criterion for distinguishing benign from malignant disease. Intact lobules are occasionally seen in aspirates from palpable breast lesions as well as in specimens obtained by stereotaxis.

The rest of the breast between the lobules and

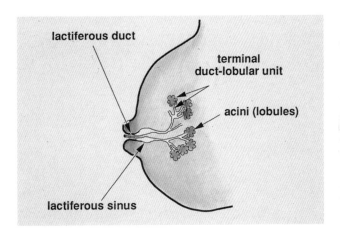

Figure 2.1 This schematic diagram of a section through the breast illustrates the terminal duct lobular units which become continuous with the lactiferous ducts.

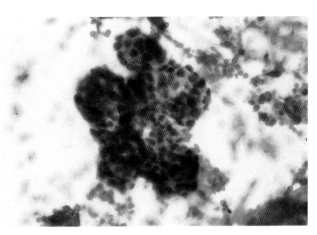

Figure 2.2 Cytology – normal breast. This low-power field of a fine needle aspirate shows a collection of small lobular or acinar units surrounded by fat cells (Pap).

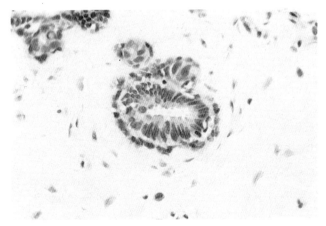

Figure 2.3 Histology – normal duct. This section shows a duct lined by two layers of cells, the inner one composed of ductal cells with an outer layer of myoepithelial cells (H & E).

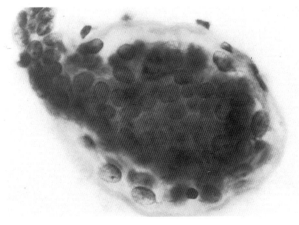

Figure 2.4 Cytology – normal duct. A high-power field which shows a sheet of small uniform benign ductal cells surrounded by a layer of loosely cohesive myoepithelial cells (Pap).

ducts is occupied by fatty stromal connective tissue. This varies in denseness depending on whether it is at an interlobular site or elsewhere in the breast but it is never very cellular. A fine needle aspirate taken from the non-pregnant, non-lactating breast is therefore sparsely cellular and composed of fragments of connective tissue and mature fat cells, the latter occasionally traversed by capillaries, with perhaps an occasional cluster of benign epithelial cells (Fig. 2.4). Using the criteria usually applied to fine needle aspirates for adequacy of the sample (an inadequate sample is one in which there are less than five clumps of epithelial cells) [1] an aspirate from the normal breast would therefore frequently fall into the 'inadequate' category.

GENERAL CYTOLOGICAL INDICATORS OF BENIGNITY

Cells aspirated from benign lesions show good cohesion and tend to form flat single-layered sheets which may show branching. These sheets can show the 'honeycombing' effect commonly seen in endocervical cells. Sometimes, especially in stereotactic fine needle aspirate specimens, complete lobular structures are aspirated which retain their three-dimensional appearance. Benign clusters do not usually show an acinar arrangement which is more often seen in carcinoma.

The overall pattern shows a mixture of duct epithelial and myoepithelial cells, the latter recognizable as single nuclei without cytoplasm ('sentinel' cells, 'naked' nuclei) or bipolar nuclei. Also present are more pointed spindle-shaped nuclei which are probably stromal in origin as well as the ubiquitous foamy macrophage. Apocrine cells and fat cells are commonly present in benign aspirates, as are fatty stromal fragments. Inflammatory cells are not unique to benign lesions, nor are foamy macrophages and multinucleated giant histiocytes.

Epithelial cells from the breast show the usual features of benignity such as uniformity of appearance (monomorphism) and size (the nucleus of a benign ductal cell is approximately twice the size of an erythrocyte). The nuclear-cytoplasmic ratio however, is high in benign ductal cells so this is not a reliable criterion for differentiating benign from malignant cells. The nucleus is round or oval with a smooth sharp nuclear margin. The chromatin pattern is vesicular or finely reticular and a small single nucleolus may be apparent. All these nuclear features are more clearly discernible on wet-fixed smears stained by the Papanicolaou method. Mitotic figures may be seen very occasionally in benign, active lesions particularly fibroadenoma but they are never abnormal.

The background in cytological samples can be important. For example, a lipid-rich background is a reassuring feature denoting lactational changes when slightly enlarged dissociated cells are present in the smear. Necrotic debris is not a feature of benign conditions but granular debris is commonly seen in cyst deposits and aspirates from duct ectasia.

PREGNANCY AND LACTATIONAL CHANGES

During pregnancy and lactation the lobules in the breast proliferate and both the acinar cells of the lobules and the ductal cells show secretory changes. In the last three months of pregnancy fat droplets accumulate within the cytoplasm of the epithelial cells (Fig. 2.5). Fine needle aspirates from the breast of a pregnant or lactating woman show a lipid-rich secretory background with small clusters of slightly enlarged epithelial cells (Fig. 2.6). The bubbly background is more obvious in air-dried, May–Grünwald Giemsa-stained smears (Fig. 2.7). The cellularity of these aspirates is variable. The cells often have conspicuous nucleoli indicative of increased activity and finely vacuolated cytoplasm, with some degree of dissociation (Fig. 2.8). There may be some nuclear enlargement and mild pleomorphism [2]. These aspirates may sometimes closely mimic carcinoma

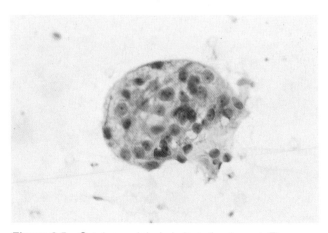

Figure 2.5 Cytology – lobule in lactating breast. The lobule illustrated in this photo-micrograph is enlarged and distended with epithelial cells containing prominent nucleoli and secretion (Pap).

and careful attention must be paid to the secretory background, normal vesicular chromatin pattern and the presence of myoepithelial cells to prevent misdiagnosis.

Focal lactational-type changes have been reported in non-pregnant, non-lactating women [3], associated with the use of hormones, antipsychotic drugs and anti-hypertensive treatment [4]. Fibroadenomas and juvenile fibroadenomas may also show focal lactational changes in pregnancy [5].

Lactating adenoma

Lactating adenomas form discrete mobile non-tender breast lumps. Histologically the entity comprises small ducts showing secretory changes (Fig. 2.9). They may arise in a pre-existing lobular adenoma. Aspirates from a lactating adenoma are highly cellular with a background rich in lipid droplets and granular material. The epithelial cells are present in large spherical, three-dimensional clusters maintain-

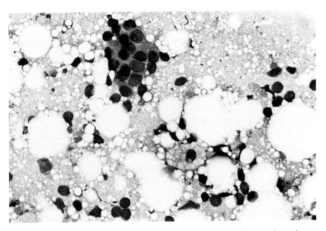

Figure 2.6 Cytology – lactational changes. Lactational changes include enlargement of the epithelial cells with some loss of cohesion, foamy cytoplasm and prominent nucleoli (Pap).

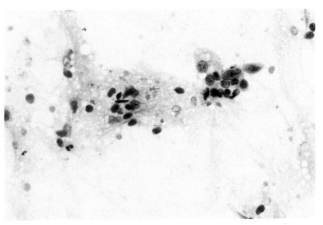

Figure 2.7 Cytology – lactational changes. The background in an aspirate from a breast showing lactational changes often has a bubbly appearance with some granular material, best appreciated in the air-dried smear (MGG).

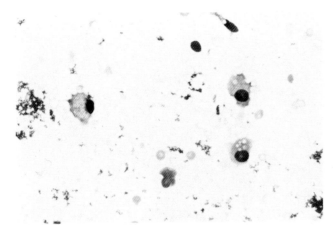

Figure 2.8 Cytology – lactational changes. Another feature which accompanies lactational change is cell dissociation. The enlarged single cells have foamy cytoplasm and may be wrongly interpreted as malignant cells (MGG).

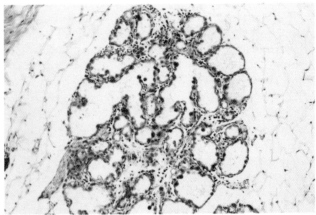

Figure 2.9 Histology – lactating adenoma. This section shows a closely packed collection of acini exhibiting cellular secretory changes as well as secretory material within the lumina of the acini (H & E).

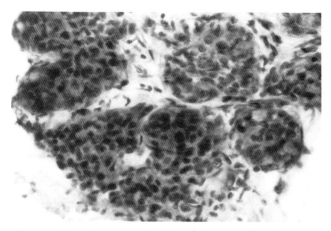

Figure 2.10 Cytology – lactating adenoma. The fine needle aspirate from a lactating adenoma shows numerous enlarged lobular structures containing epithelial cells with prominent nucleoli. Some myoepithelial cells are seen in the background (Pap). Compare this with the normal lobule in Fig. 2.2.

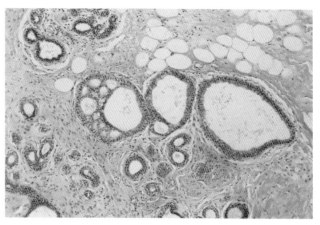

Figure 2.11 Histology – benign proliferative breast changes. This section of breast shows proliferative and cystic changes with no evidence of malignancy (H & E). Courtesy of Dr M. Cook.

ing normal lobular architecture [6] (Fig. 2.10), and contain abundant vacuolated cytoplasm. Nucleoli are visible though not greatly enlarged. The clusters of epithelial cells are surrounded by myoepithelial cells [7].

BENIGN PROLIFERATIVE CHANGES

As the breast matures various proliferative [8] and degenerative changes occur that may form focal lesions (Fig. 2.11) and these have been given a variety of names including fibrocystic disease, fibroadenosis, and benign mastopathy amongst others. The terminology of benign breast pathology has been a controversial issue [9] and it has been suggested that a better name may be Aberrations of Normal Development and Involution (ANDI) [10] in order to provide a term that removes the stigma of a 'disease' but provides a name based on the probable pathogenesis of such lesions. Aspirates are more cellular than those from the normal breast. They contain flat sheets of small, uniform benign ductal cells with rounded or oval vesicular nuclei, often containing visible nucleoli. The nuclei usually do not overlap. The nuclear-cytoplasmic ratio is high in benign ductal cells as they have little cytoplasm (Fig. 2.4). Many myoepithelial cells are seen. These appear in the form of bipolar or torpedo-shaped

nuclei without cytoplasm which are hyperchromatic and often seen in pairs. Some controversy exists as to the origin of these naked nuclei, one school of thought believing them to represent stromal cells and the other myoepithelial cells. On careful examination both myoepithelial cells with their plump oval-to-bipolar nuclei and spindle-shaped stromal cells with their more pointed nuclei and wisps of cytoplasm are seen in benign aspirates (Figs 2.12, 2.13). Stromal fragments are present showing various degrees of cellularity. In wet-fixed, Papanicolaou-stained smears they stain pale blue-green (Fig. 2.14) while in air-dried smears they stain a vivid pinkish purple (Fig. 2.15).

Blunt duct adenosis cannot be identified with certainty in aspirates. Sclerosing adenosis which is a change in the structure of the lobule (Fig. 2.16) is represented in aspirates by thick clusters of small epithelial cells with superimposed bare bipolar myoepithelial cell nuclei (Fig. 2.17). This is in marked contrast to the normal lobules (see Fig. 2.2) with their outer lining of myoepithelial cells. Apocrine cell change associated with sclerosing adenosis may be mistaken for carcinoma [1]. Again the presence of myoepithelial cells is a reassuring feature.

The term 'adenosis tumour' is used to describe a breast lesion composed of localized sclerosing adenosis changes presenting as a palpable mass. Fine needle aspiration cytology reveals fragments of

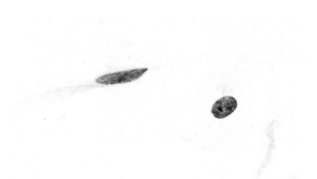

Figure 2.12 Cytology – bare nuclei. The origin of the bare nuclei seen in benign aspirates is greatly disputed. This field shows a myoepithelial cell nucleus which is oval, and a thin pointed stromal cell nucleus indicating that both types of cells are present (Pap).

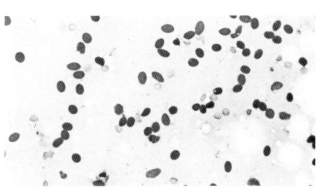

Figure 2.13 Cytology – bare nuclei. Many myoepithelial cell nuclei, some apparently in groups of two or three. The nuclei are plump and oval as opposed to spindle-shaped stromal nuclei (MGG).

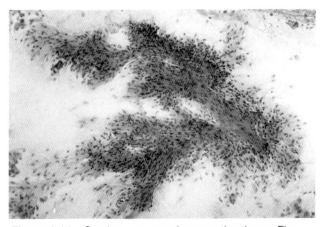

Figure 2.14 Cytology – stromal connective tissue. Fine needle aspirates often contain large stromal fragments varying in cellularity from poor to hypercellular as in this case. The fibroblasts within the fragments have pointed spindle-shaped nuclei (Pap).

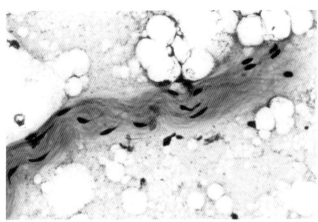

Figure 2.15 Same as Fig. 2.14 stained with MGG.

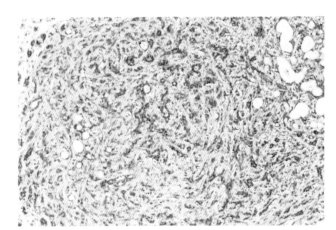

Figure 2.16 Histology – sclerosing adenosis. This section shows lobules compressed by swirling streams of myoepithelial cells. On a frozen section the appearances can mimic malignancy (H & E).

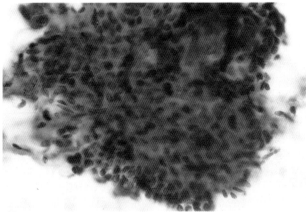

Figure 2.17 Cytology – sclerosing adenosis. A fine needle aspirate from an area of sclerosing adenosis shows a thick cluster of small epithelial cells with scattered myoepithelial cells. Some calcium is also present (arrow) (Pap).

hyalinized stroma with spindle cells, sheets of benign ductal cells and numerous bare nuclei. It cannot be differentiated cytologically from other benign proliferative lesions [11].

Ductal hyperplasia is represented in aspirates by three-dimensional clusters of slightly enlarged benign ductal cells accompanied by myoepithelial cells. Although the nuclei overlap somewhat there is no nuclear pleomorphism (Fig. 2.18). Aspirates from areas of atypical epithelial hyperplasia can be moderately or abundantly cellular with sheets of epithelial cells showing some nuclear enlargement and overlapping, conspicuous nucleoli and a finely granular chromatin pattern (Fig. 2.19). The epithelial changes are more severe than in ordinary hyperplasia and although myoepithelial cells are usually present the picture may warrant a 'suspicious' report. Occasionally apocrine cells and foamy macrophages are also seen. Atypical lobular hyperplasia cannot be reliably diagnosed on aspirates.

RADIAL SCAR/COMPLEX SCLEROSING LESION

With the advent of mammographic screening and the rapidly expanding use of stereotactic techniques, smaller breast lesions are being sampled for cytological assessment (see also Chapter 8). One such type of mammographic abnormality, namely the small stellate or spiculate lesion, can cause diagnostic problems for both radiologist and pathologist alike. Mammographically such a lesion may represent either a radial scar/complex sclerosing lesion or a tubular carcinoma (Fig. 2.20) and furthermore it has been suggested that tubular carcinomas are possibly derived from radial scars [12]. Histologically the centre of a radial scar is composed of dense fibroelastotic tissue with a few trapped ductules while the periphery exhibits varying degrees of epithelial hyperplasia which is sometimes atypical (Fig. 2.21).

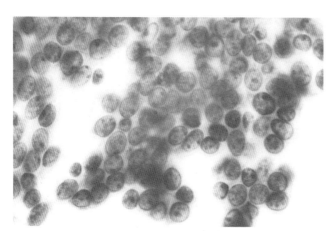

Figure 2.18 Cytology – simple ductal hyperplasia. In simple ductal hyperplasia the epithelial cells remain uniform although their nuclei may be slightly enlarged and show a minor degree of overlapping compared with the flat sheets of ductal cells seen in a fibroadenoma, for example, see Fig. 2.42 (Pap).

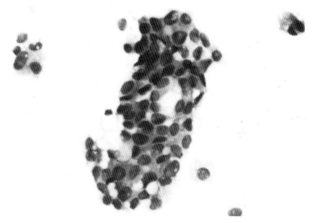

Figure 2.19 Cytology – atypical ductal hyperplasia. This air-dried smear shows more marked nuclear variation than is seen in a wet-fixed smear (MGG).

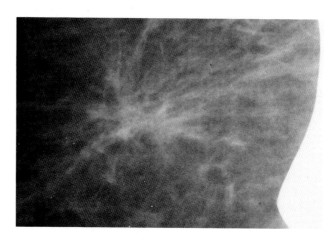

Figure 2.20 Mammogram of radial scar. Within this fatty breast there is an irregular stellate density with spiculated margins. Long thin strands of tissue radiate circumferentially around an irregular central core. Radiologically it is not possible to differentiate between a benign condition such as a radial scar or a small scirrhous or tubular carcinoma. Cytology is helpful only if it confirms malignancy, when definitive surgery can be performed. Even if cytology is benign, surgical removal of stellate abnormalities is recommended for definitive histological analysis. Courtesy of Dr Julie Cooke.

Stereotactic fine needle aspirates are usually sparsely or moderately cellular showing sheets of benign ductal cells, some myoepithelial cells and stromal fragments. If the aspirate has been taken from a hyperplastic area the epithelial cells appear in smaller, rounded, loosely cohesive clusters and show nuclear enlargement, mild pleomorphism and conspicuous nucleoli. Myoepithelial cells are often scanty. This type of aspirate may have to be reported as 'suspicious' because of the uncertain nature of the appearances (Fig. 2.22). In a case where histopathological biopsy showed atypical ductal hyperplasia when the aspirate (Fig. 2.23) showed typical malignant cells, further sections at deeper level revealed ductal carcinoma *in situ*.

In the author's experience of 183 stellate lesions detected mammographically (Table 2.1), all 47 cases reported as C5 (carcinoma) were malignant on histology. Twenty-six of the 40 cases reported as suspicious (C3, C4) were also malignant on biopsy and 18 of 50 cases reported benign (C2) showed carcinoma on histology illustrating why all spiculate lesions should be surgically removed. Some spiculate lesions which have been present for years are being followed up mammographically rather than biopsied.

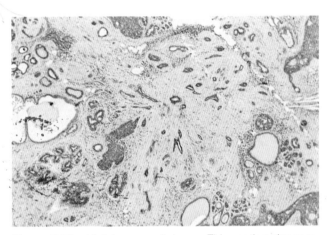

Figure 2.21 Histology – radial scar. This section shows a lesion with a fibroelastotic centre containing trapped tubules and radiating proliferative areas (H & E).

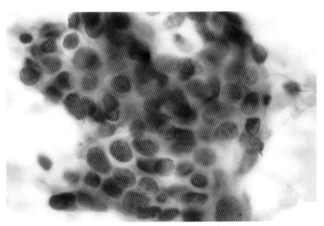

Figure 2.22 Cytology – radial scar. A cluster of epithelial cells which are variable in nuclear size with distinct nucleoli and clumped chromatin. Although the appearances are not diagnostic of carcinoma, they are highly suspicious (Pap).

Table 2.1   Cytology and histology of 183 mammographic stellate breast lesions

	Histology			
	Benign	Atypical ductal hyperplasia	Malignant	Not available/ not done
Cytology inadequate, C1	7	0	20	19
Cytology benign, C2	17	3	18	12
Cytology suspicious, C3/C4	4	9	26	1
Cytology malignant, C5	0	0	47	0
Totals	28	12	111	32

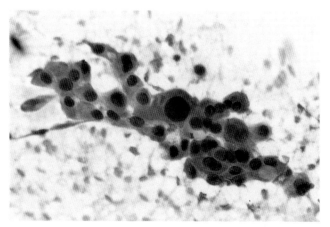

Figure 2.23 Cytology – ductal carcinoma *in situ*. A cluster of cohesive but enlarged pleomorphic ductal cells suggestive of carcinoma. Biopsy revealed atypical ductal hyperplasia which on further sectioning was found to be continuous with ductal carcinoma *in situ* (MGG).

DUCT ECTASIA

This condition may present clinically as a palpable central mass but it is an incidental finding in its early stages. It is due to dilated ducts which appear on mammographs as wormlike structures (Fig. 2.24) and it is commonly associated with a surrounding inflammatory infiltrate in which plasma cells sometimes predominate (Fig. 2.25). Large ducts, usually those near the areola, become distended with amorphous material admixed with foamy macrophages (Fig. 2.26). The pressure caused by the contents of the ducts flattens the lining ductal epithelium so an aspirate from such an area shows debris and numerous foamy macrophages but usually no epithelial cells (Fig. 2.27). Although there is often periductal inflammation justifying the other name for this condition – plasma cell mastitis [13] – inflammatory cells are rarely seen in aspirates. Because of the location of this lesion near the areola, nipple discharge is often a feature. The nipple discharge smear shows debris and foamy macrophages.

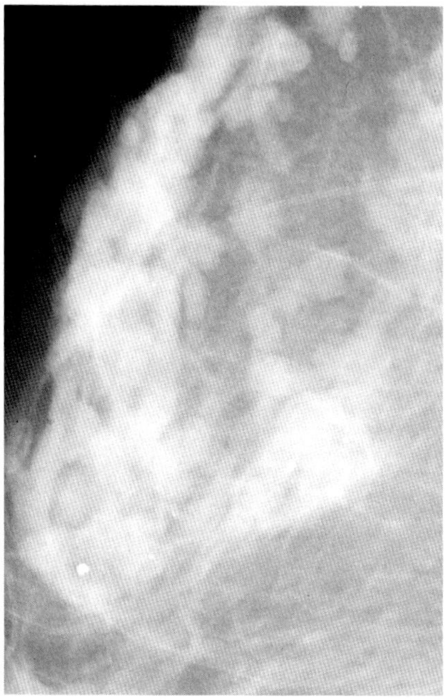

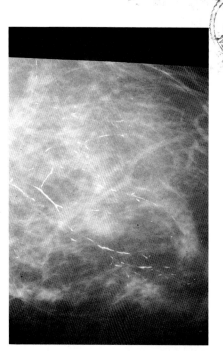

Figure 2.24 Mammogram showing dilated ducts. Dilated ducts in this predominantly fatty breast show as tubular wormlike structures extending from the nipple towards the axillary tail. It is unusual to see normal ducts on a mammogram. Asymmetric duct dilatation can be seen with an intraductal papilloma, with a carcinoma which causes obstruction of proximal ducts, or in duct ectasia where appearances are due to stagnant duct secretions. Courtesy of Dr Julie Cooke.

Figure 2.25 Mammogram showing 'plasma cell mastitis'. The calcifications in this mammogram have the typical appearance of 'plasma cell mastitis'. The particles lie within the duct lumen and conform to the shape of the ducts. They are well-defined with a crisp outline and a linear, occasionally branching shape, radiating towards the nipple along the line of the ducts. Courtesy of Dr Julie Cooke.

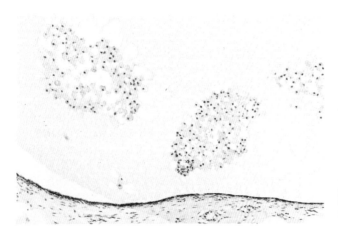

Figure 2.26 Histology – duct ectasia. This section shows part of the wall of a dilated duct lined by flattened epithelial cells. The lumen contains clumps of foamy macrophages (H & E).

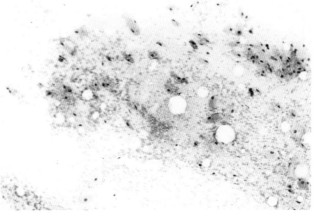

Figure 2.27 Cytology – duct ectasia. This illustrates a background of granular debris and foamy macrophages characteristic of these aspirates (MGG).

BREAST CYSTS

Breast cysts are usually found in women between the ages of 50 and 65 years [14]. Some women are more prone to develop them than others. Cysts show up on mammograms (Fig. 2.28) and especially on ultrasound examination when their cystic nature can be demonstrated (Fig. 2.29). They vary in size and fluid volume and have been shown to disappear on post-aspiration mammograms. Cyst fluid which is transparent and runny is invariably benign and can be discarded by the clinician. Ciatto *et al.* [15] reviewed the results of cytological examination of 6782 cyst fluids from 4105 women and concluded that all significant lesions unsuspected clinically, produced blood-stained fluid. Breast cyst fluid which is discoloured, whether blood-stained, brown, green or thick in consistency should always

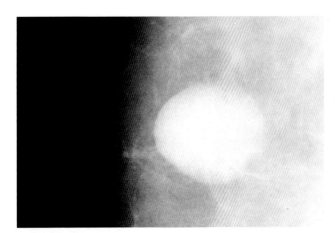

Figure 2.28 Mammogram of a cyst. There is a round dense well-defined mass lying close to the skin surface. Mammographically it is impossible to determine whether this lesion is solid or whether it contains fluid. A non-invasive means of differentiating a cyst from a solid carcinoma or fibroadenoma is by using diagnostic ultrasound. Courtesy of Dr Julie Cooke.

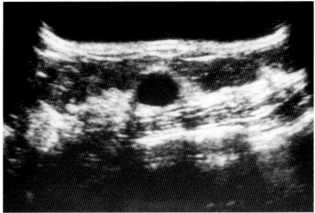

Figure 2.29 Ultrasound of a cyst. Lying beneath the skin surface is a well-defined lesion containing no internal echoes. A simple cyst is the only circumscribed ultrasound abnormality which is completely echo-free. The presence of a well-defined posterior wall and a 'bright shadow' behind the lesion are also characteristic features. Courtesy of Dr Julie Cooke.

be sent for cytological examination. Fluid should also be sent for assessment if there is a residual mass after aspiration or if it is from a recurrent cyst. Fluid should be collected in a clean universal container and sent to the laboratory where the specimen is centrifuged and the spun deposit examined.

Benign cysts contain granular debris, altered blood (when the fluid is often dark brown), many foamy macrophages and sometimes some polymorphonuclear leucocytes (Fig. 2.30). Some of the foamy macrophages appear to be derived from the clusters of benign epithelial cells that are usually seen in the sample. These epithelial cells may appear in the form of flat sheets or rounded clusters often with cytoplasmic changes resembling that of foamy macrophages towards the edges of the cluster (Fig. 2.31). Other foamy macrophages are true histiocytes. They have rounded or bean-shaped nuclei with a sharp nuclear margin, a noticeable nucleolus and foamy, finely vacuolated cytoplasm. In the wet-fixed, Papanicolaou-stained smear, pink intracytoplasmic inclusion bodies may be observed. These are believed to be large lysosomes which develop as a result of the phagocytic activity of macrophages [16]. Occasionally slight cellular atypia is seen in the form of nuclear enlargement accompanied by degenerative changes such as loss of sharp nuclear outlines and cytoplasmic vacuolation (Fig. 2.32). This atypia should not be mistaken for neoplasia. Sheets of apocrine cells are a frequent feature. They are large cells with abundant cytoplasm, eccentric nuclei, prominent nucleoli and cytoplasmic granules which show up more clearly on the air-dried smear stained with May–Grünwald Giemsa than on the wet-fixed,

Papanicolaou-stained smear (Figs 2.33, 2.34). Much debris resembling the granular material in apocrine cells is seen in cyst fluid smears. However, necrotic cellular debris is never seen in benign cysts and if present should always prompt a thorough search for malignant cells from an intracystic carcinoma. Calcification is occasionally seen in cyst fluids (Fig. 2.35). On occasions cells are seen which contain large nuclei with prominent nucleoli and plentiful cyanophilic cytoplasm, which appear almost spindle-shaped. These represent fibroblasts from the inflammatory granulation tissue which occasionally surrounds cysts (Fig. 2.36).

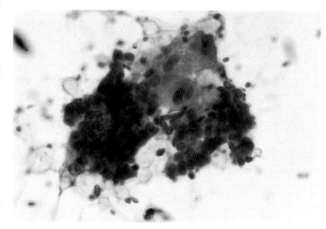

Figure 2.31 Cytology – breast cyst fluid. Some of the cells at the periphery of the cluster of epithelial cells apparently take on a histiocytic appearance with vacuolated cytoplasm (Pap).

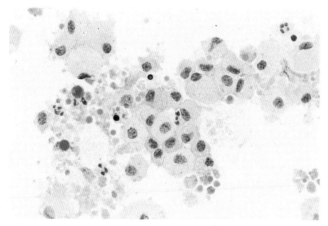

Figure 2.30 Cytology – breast cyst fluid. Foamy macrophages with their delicate cytoplasm and eccentric nuclei are a typical feature of benign breast cysts. Occasionally multinucleated giant hystiocytes are seen (MGG).

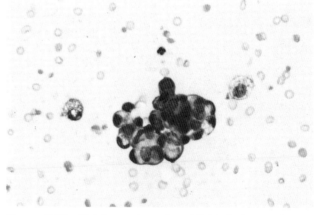

Figure 2.32 Cytology – breast cyst fluid. A cluster of degenerate ductal cells exhibiting vacuolation. This should not be mistaken for malignancy. Note the foamy macrophages in the background (MGG).

GALACTOCOELE

The accumulation of milk secretion in ducts may be large enough to produce a palpable swelling. The mammographic appearances are typical (Fig. 2.37). Aspiration reveals background material containing bubbly lipid secretions with epithelial cells showing secretory vacuolation.

FIBROADENOMA

Fibroadenomas are discrete proliferative biphasic lesions composed of both stromal and epithelial elements (Fig. 2.38). They present clinically as rounded mobile palpable masses, fancifully termed 'breast mice', which may be difficult to localize while being aspirated. Mammography can detect impalp-

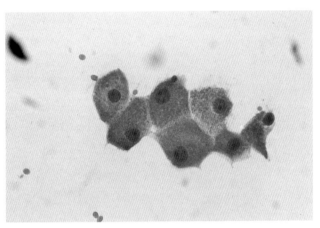

Figure 2.33 Cytology – breast cyst fluid. Apocrine cells are seen in flat sheets. Note the abundant granular cytoplasm, large eccentric nuclei and prominent nucleoli. Occasional cells are binucleate. There is debris in the background (Pap).

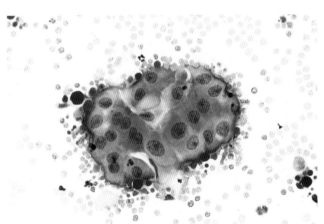

Figure 2.34 Cytology – breast cyst fluid. Apocrine cells stain purple with the MGG stain. The large nuclei with their enormous nucleoli often pose a problem to the beginner as they are mistaken for malignancy. Occasional cells are binucleate. Note the cyst debris in the background (MGG).

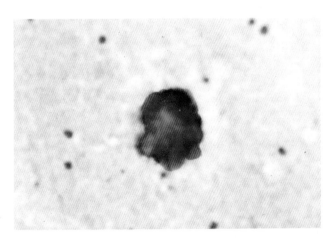

Figure 2.35 Breast cyst fluid. Calcium is rarely seen in breast cyst fluid. In the wet-fixed smear it appears as irregular chunks of deep pink to red material (Pap).

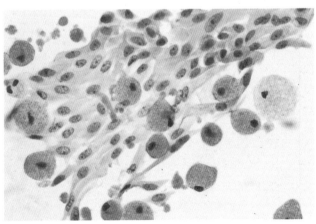

Figure 2.36 Breast cyst fluid. A mixture of foamy macrophages and spindle-shaped cells with abundant cytoplasm and prominent nucleoli, believed to be fibroblasts, is present (Pap).

able fibroadenomas which also tend to have a rubbery, bouncy feel on stereotactic aspiration. Mammographically a fibroadenoma appears as a well-demarcated rounded lesion (Fig. 2.39).

Fine needle aspirates from these lesions vary in cellularity depending upon the amount and denseness of the stroma. Usually the aspirate is cellular, especially those from young women, containing large, sometimes enormous flat sheets of small uniform benign ductal cells. A feature often seen is the 'antler-horn' branching effect of some of the sheets of epithelial cells (Fig. 2.40). Sometimes the branches are club-shaped (Fig. 2.41). The margins of the sheets are usually smooth and the cells cohesive. Very large ductal sheets are often folded (Fig. 2.42). Sprinkled over the epithelial cells are small hyper-

chromatic bare bipolar nuclei – myoepithelial cells. These are best seen in wet-fixed aspirates (Fig. 2.43) like sesame seeds scattered over a loaf of bread. These bare nuclei are also seen in large numbers in the background. On the basis of ultrasound studies it has been shown that most of the bare nuclei in aspirates are stromal cells [17], although many do resemble myoepithelial cells. The third typical feature seen in fibroadenoma aspirates is the presence of fragments of connective tissue stroma. These vary in cellularity, showing spindle-shaped fibroblasts in a myxoid-type matrix which stains pale pink or blue in the wet-fixed preparation and bright purplish-pink in the air-dried smear (Figs 2.14, 2.15). The ductal cells in the sheets often have conspicuous nucleoli which are a feature indicative of actively

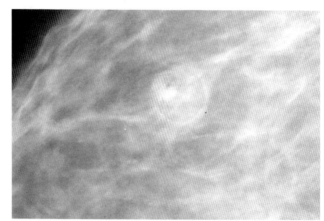

Figure 2.37 Mammogram – galactocoele. A galactocoele usually occurs during or just after lactation. A build-up of secretions occurs and a cystic structure forms which is situated close to the nipple. Saponification of milk occurs. On a mammogram a galactocoele appears as a round mass containing low-density fatty material separated from a dense component which represents semisolid milk. Courtesy of Dr Julie Cooke.

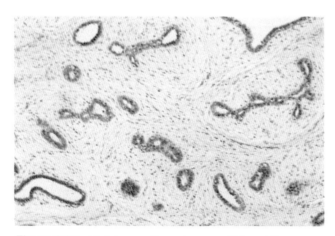

Figure 2.38 Histology – fibroadenoma. This section shows a typical pericanalicular fibroadenoma (H & E).

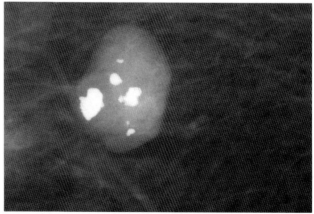

Figure 2.39 Mammogram – fibroadenoma. This mammogram shows an oval, slightly lobulated, well-defined soft tissue mass containing coarse irregular calcification particles. Popcorn calcification seen in association with a soft tissue mass is characteristic of a hyalinizing fibroadenoma. Courtesy of Dr Julie Cooke.

growing fibroadenomas, as are mitotic figures. However, the chromatin pattern is always vesicular and the nuclear outlines smooth and rounded (Fig. 2.44). Apocrine cells are seen frequently, as are foamy macrophages. The cells seen reflect the histological patterns, although it is not possible to tell from the cytology whether a fibroadenoma is of pericanalicular or intracanalicular type.

It has been noted that while wet-fixed aspirates tend to contain typical cohesive sheets of benign ductal cells often the air-dried smears from the same aspirate show some epithelial cell dissociation making interpretation difficult (Fig. 2.45). It is thus useful to have both types of preparations for comparison.

Whereas histological sections of fibroadenomas frequently show focal atypia, fine needle aspirates rarely show corresponding changes, possibly due to inadequate sampling [18]. It has been postulated that atypical epithelial proliferation and marked secretory activity in fibroadenomas may be linked to oral contraceptive usage [19]. The histological atypia

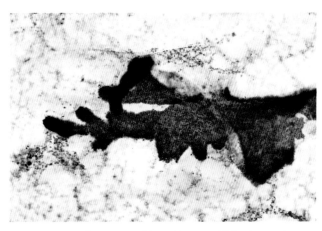

Figure 2.40 Cytology – fibroadenoma. This sheet of benign ductal cells exhibits the typical stag-horn or antler-horn branching seen in fibroadenomas (Pap).

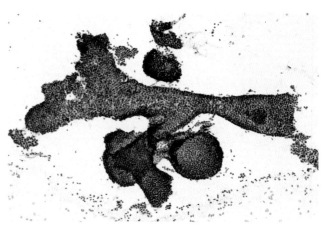

Figure 2.41 Cytology – fibroadenoma. Ductal sheets with blunt club-shaped branches are another feature often seen in fibroadenomas. Note the bare nuclei in the background (Pap).

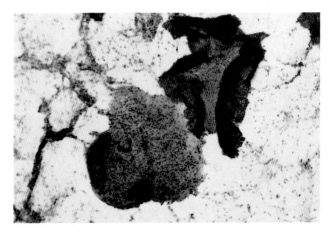

Figure 2.42 Cytology – fibroadenoma. A large sheet of benign ductal cells with its edges folded over and a scattering of myoepithelial cells over its surface like sesame seeds over a loaf of bread. Note the large fragment of cellular connective tissue adjacent to ductal cells (Pap).

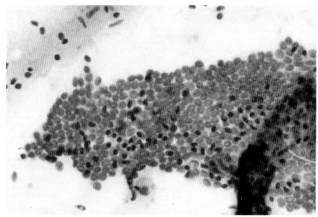

Figure 2.43 Cytology – fibroadenoma. The ductal cells are in a cohesive sheet with scattered bare nuclei in the background, a mixture of myoepithelial and stromal cells (Pap).

is reflected in the aspirate as sheets of enlarged epithelial cells with hyperchromatic, mildly pleomorphic nuclei. These cells are often part of a sheet which in other areas is composed of small, uniform, typical benign ductal cells (Fig. 2.46). The presence of scattered bare nuclei is a helpful feature in ruling out carcinoma. These can be confirmed as myoepithelial cells by using the antiserum CALLA (the common acute lymphoblastic leukaemia antigen) [20] and myoepithelial actin can also be demonstrated immunocytochemically. It has been sug-

gested that the cyclical hormonal changes related to endometrial activity may be responsible for the atypia that is occasionally seen in fibroadenomas [18].

Another pitfall in the interpretation of aspirates from fibroadenomas is the presence of myxoid or mucinous-type material in the background which may be highly suggestive of mucinous carcinoma [21] (Fig. 2.47). In such carcinomas the malignant cells are often well-differentiated and in cohesive groups making it particularly easy to falsely diag-

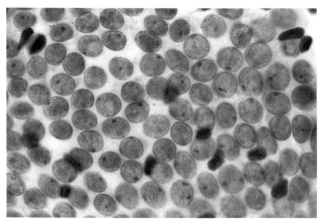

Figure 2.44 Cytology – fibroadenoma. A high-power view of benign ductal cells shows their smooth rounded nuclear outlines, vesicular chromatin pattern and visible nucleoli (Pap).

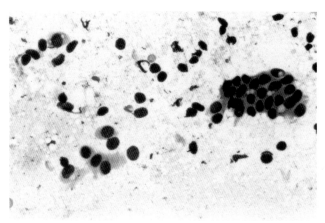

Figure 2.45 Cytology – fibroadenoma. A sheet of benign ductal cells as well as some dissociated cells in the background. This seems to be a peculiarity of air-dried smears (MGG).

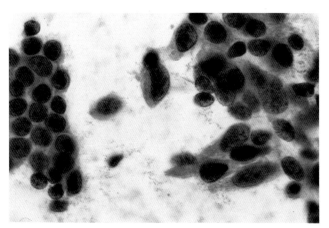

Figure 2.46 Cytology – atypical fibroadenoma. On the left note the orderly arrangement of small uniform ductal cells. On the right the cells are pleomorphic and appear to be dissociating. This is a pitfall which can be avoided by searching for bare nuclei and noting that in areas some of the pleomorphic cells are attached to sheets of benign ductal cells (Pap).

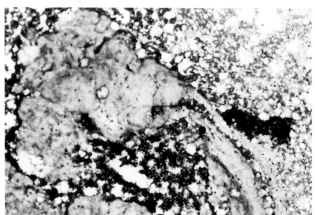

Figure 2.47 Cytology – mucin in fibroadenomas. Stromal myxoid material may rarely be seen in aspirates from fibroadenomas. A careful search must be made for malignant cells to exclude the possibility of a mucinous carcinoma (MGG).

nose fibroadenomas. This mistake may occur in stereotactic aspirates also, as mucinous carcinomas can show on mammograms as lobulated, fairly well-circumscribed densities similar to fibroadenomas. However, the lesion usually feels rubbery to the tip of the needle in a fibroadenoma and also the presence of myoepithelial cells is a pointer to the benign nature of the aspirate [22].

Proliferation of the glandular component of a fibroadenoma may be so extensive as to produce a highly cellular aspirate with epithelial cells showing mild pleomorphism (Fig. 2.48) and a histological picture almost amounting to tubular adenoma (Fig. 2.49).

Fibroadenomas may show focal lactational changes [4]. The cells aspirated from such areas show secretory vacuolation of their cytoplasm and prominent nucleoli with some cell dissociation but here again the presence of bipolar nuclei is helpful in arriving at the correct diagnosis.

INFLAMMATORY CONDITIONS OF THE BREAST

Mastitis

Acute mastitis is clinically obvious with pain, redness, swelling and tenderness over the affected area of the breast and is not usually aspirated. A course of antibiotics clears the condition but occasionally a mass remains in the breast which is non-tender,

representing chronic mastitis. A fine needle aspirate from an area of chronic mastitis is extremely cellular containing many foamy macrophages, multinucleated giant histiocytes, polymorphonuclear leucocytes and background debris (Fig. 2.50). Clusters of benign epithelial cells are seen which may show some atypia, namely nuclear enlargement or degenerative changes such as cytoplasmic vacuolation (Fig. 2.51).

Subareolar abscess

This is a special type of recurring low-grade infection of the subareolar region. An aspirate will show an identical cytological picture to that of chronic mastitis with the addition of keratinized anucleate squames as a consequence of the squamous metaplasia that occurs in the nipple ducts. The squamous cells stain a bright refractile orange with the Papanicolaou stain (Fig. 2.52) and a dense sky-blue colour with the May–Grünwald Giemsa stain (Fig. 2.53).

Granulomatous mastitis

This uncommon entity is characterized by a granulomatous inflammatory process composed of epithelioid histiocytes, Langhans-type giant cells and chronic inflammatory cells in lobular areas of the breast (Fig. 2.54) [23]. Clinically the patients are usually young and the condition may be mistaken for a

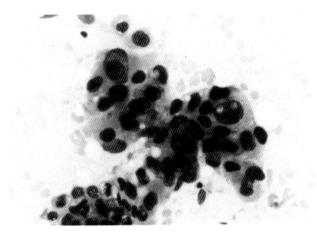

Figure 2.48 Cytology – fibroadenoma. The air-dried smear accentuates the pleomorphism in this case but the rest of the smear showed many sheets of benign ductal cells and myoepithelial cells (MGG).

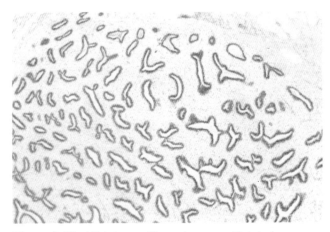

Figure 2.49 Histology – fibroadenoma with tubular adenoma-like changes. Part of an atypical fibroadenoma which shows an area of tubular adenoma-like change with numerous small tubules (H & E).

carcinoma. The disease follows a prolonged course in some patients sometimes necessitating several operations. In the absence of a microbiological cause the aetiology is uncertain but an autoimmune process is possibly involved and there may be an ischaemic component in the pathogenesis. Other theories which have been suggested include squamous metaplasia with keratin products stimulating a foreign body reaction, also blocked secretions secondary to increased secretory activity due to either oral contraceptive use or the presence of a pituitary tumour [24].

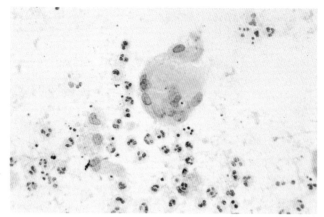

Figure 2.50 Cytology – mastitis. Note the multinucleated giant histiocytes, small histiocytes and polymorphs in this aspirate from a focus of chronic mastitis (Pap).

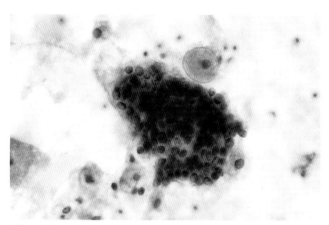

Figure 2.51 Cytology – mastitis. The sheet of benign ductal cells seen here shows some cytoplasmic vacuolation but no evidence of malignancy. Note the foamy macrophages in the background (Pap).

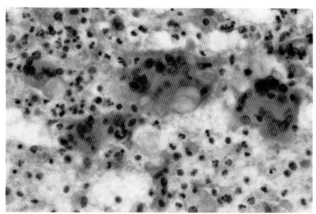

Figure 2.52 Cytology – sub-areolar abscess. The cytological appearances are similar to those seen in mastitis with multinucleated giant cells, histiocytes and polymorphs. However, note the pale orange anucleate squames in the background (Pap).

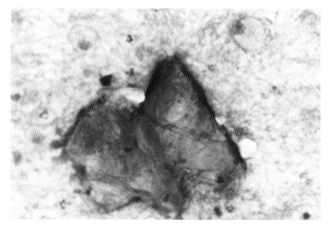

Figure 2.53 Cytology – sub-areolar abscess. Keratinized anucleate squames stain a striking shade of azure blue with the May–Grunwald Giemsa stain, and are therefore much more easily identified than in a Papanicolaou–stained smear (MGG).

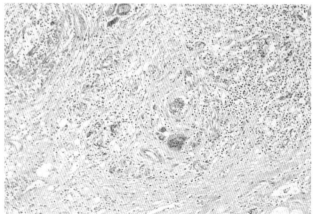

Figure 2.54 Histology – granulomatous mastitis. Scattered granulomas composed of Langhans-type giant cells and inflammatory cells (H & E).

In the Indian subcontinent a high proportion of inflammatory breast lesions have a tuberculous aetiology with the typical cytological features of granulomatous mastitis [25]. An uncommon infectious agent producing the characteristic cytologic appearance of granulomatous mastitis is histoplasma [26].

Aspiration cytology shows foamy macrophages, footprint-shaped epithelioid histiocytes, proliferative blood vessels, multinucleated giant histiocytes (Fig. 2.55) and Langhans-type giant cells (Fig. 2.56). Fungal and tuberculous infections must be excluded by using special stains such as PAS and Ziehl–Neilsen, if sufficient material is available. Sarcoidosis may produce a similar cytological picture while in silicon granuloma vacuoles of various sizes within histiocytes are seen [27].

Fat necrosis

Cytology is a very useful diagnostic tool in this condition which presents as a hard irregular mass in the breast, often clinically indistinguishable from carcinoma (Fig. 2.57). A history of trauma may be elicited on careful questioning but there is sometimes quite a long interval between the trauma and the development of symptoms and the injury is often forgotten. Mammography is helpful in excluding carcinoma (Fig. 2.58).

Aspirates from fat necrosis show variable degrees of cellularity. Degenerate fat cells are present which quite often resemble foamy macrophages (Fig. 2.59). Inflammatory cells including polymorphs, lymphocytes, histiocytes and multinucleated histiocytes are seen. Usually no epithelial cells are evident [28].

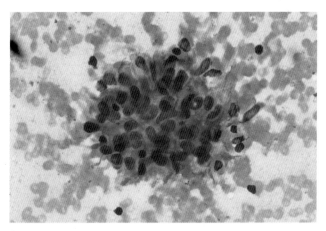

Figure 2.55 Cytology – granulomatous mastitis. This is a collection of epithelioid histiocytes with elongated footprint-shaped nuclei, associated with granulomatous mastitis. A scattering of lymphocytes is also present (MGG).

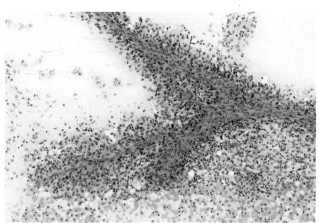

Figure 2.56 Cytology – granulomatous mastitis. This low-power field shows the proliferating capillaries often observed in aspirates from granulomatous mastitis (Pap).

Figure 2.57 Skin dimpling. This clinical photograph shows marked skin dimpling and retraction in the lower medial part of the right breast on pectoral muscle contraction. This clinical feature is highly suggestive of carcinoma, but was in fact granulomatous mastitis. Courtesy of Dr Julie Cooke.

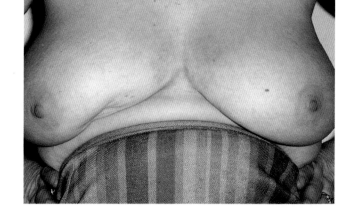

RADIATION CHANGES IN THE BREAST

Radiotherapy is frequently used in the treatment of carcinoma of the breast usually after local excision. Radiation not only destroys carcinoma cells but also produces changes in benign breast tissue which may be florid and mistaken for carcinoma in fine needle aspirates. Mammographic examination of the breast can show typical features (Fig. 2.60) but it may be unhelpful if the patient has scarring due to previous surgery and new or recurrent carcinomas may be undetectable. Cytological examination of aspirates from clinically suspicious areas is then requested.

The aspirate is often acellular, a feature which has been used to indicate benignity [29] or scanty due to post-radiation fibrosis [30], or moderately cellular,

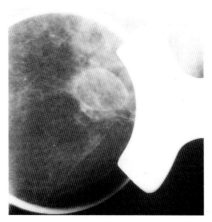

Figure 2.58 Mammogram – fat necrosis (same case as Fig. 2.57). Careful mammography of the left breast, concentrating in particular on the area beneath the dimple, did not reveal the classical signs of a carcinoma. Instead, the mammogram demonstrated a well-circumscribed mass containing low-density material. The mammographic features are consistent with a diagnosis of fat necrosis. On further questioning the patient admitted to a history of a car accident with severe bruising to the breast. Courtesy of Dr Julie Cooke.

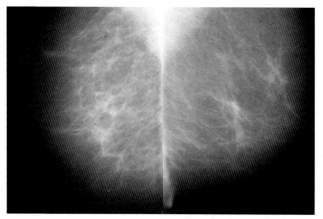

Figure 2.60 Mammogram – radiation change. Following radiotherapy in the right breast (which appears smaller than the left) there is coarsening and thickening of the breast trabeculae. The overall density of the fat is increased and there is some skin thickening. The acute changes following radiotherapy represent increased oedema which is followed by a degree of fibrosis. The changes may progress up to two years after treatment and then gradually subside and stabilize. Courtesy of Dr Julie Cooke.

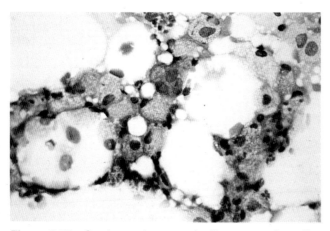

Figure 2.59 Cytology – fat necrosis. Degenerate fat cells and foamy macrophages are illustrated here suggesting a diagnosis of fat necrosis (MGG).

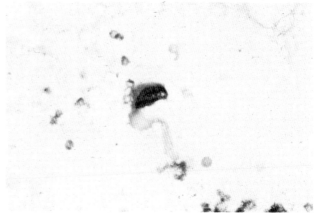

Figure 2.61 Cytology – radiation changes. This isolated cell with its enlarged nucleus mimics carcinoma but the presence of degenerative changes such as intranuclear vacuolation indicate that these changes are due to radiotherapy rather than to malignancy (Pap).

containing fragments of connective tissue and large abnormal histiocytes which are sometimes multinucleated. Occasionally there are groups of enlarged, pleomorphic hyperchromatic, nucleolated epithelial cells which may mimic carcinoma (Fig. 2.61) but true cell dissociation is not seen [31]. Degenerative changes such as vacuolation, abnormal staining and pyknosis are often features as is necrosis. Foamy macrophages may be present but few myoepithelial cells are seen. Fat necrosis has also been reported [32]. Epithelial atypia is also a feature of the irradiated breast and should not be considered indicative of carcinoma, although it has been suggested that it may sometimes represent early malignant change [33].

LIPOMA

Lipomas are clinically obvious when they are palpable as soft, fatty lumps. They may be picked up on mammography as well-demarcated translucent areas (Fig. 2.62). An aspirate from a lipoma is usually cellular, displaying large fragments of tissue composed of mature adipocytes and closely related connective tissue. No epithelial cells are seen but in the light of the clinical details this constitutes a satisfactory, benign aspirate (Fig. 2.63).

INTRAMAMMARY LYMPH NODE

Intramammary lymph nodes may occur in any part of the breast although they are usually present in the upper outer quadrant. They are seen on screening mammograms as small sharply demarcated rounded masses, often with a central clearing suggestive of fat (Fig. 2.64). Fine needle aspirates from lymph nodes are extremely cellular showing a mixed population of lymphoid cells including small lymphocytes (Fig. 2.65). It must be remembered however, that the breast is a common site for metastatic tumour and secondary malignant lymphoma must be considered in the differential diagnosis.

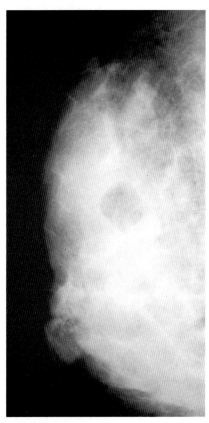

Figure 2.62 Mammogram – lipoma. This patient's breasts demonstrate a dense homogeneous mammographic pattern. Within this there is a well-defined outline of a lesion which is low in density. On a mammogram fatty tissue has a characteristic appearance and its overall density is always lower than that of glandular or fibrous tissue. This mammographic abnormality is composed entirely of fat and represents a lipoma. Courtesy of Dr Julie Cooke.

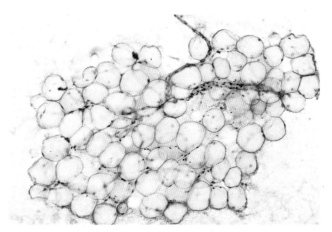

Figure 2.63 Cytology – lipoma. A large cluster of benign fat cells is seen here, traversed by a capillary. No epithelial cells are usually seen (MGG).

EPIDERMAL CYSTS

Epidermal cysts may occur in the breast, presenting as small rounded superficial lumps. They appear solid on mammography and may resemble either fibroadenomas or carcinomas. It is postulated that they originate in the breast either from residual undifferentiated basal or reserve cells or from squamous metaplasia of a simple breast cyst or fibroadenoma [34]. Recurrent epidermal cysts have been reported [35].

Histology shows a cyst lined by flattened stratified squamous epithelium including cells with cytoplasmic keratohyaline granules, containing keratin and debris (Fig. 2.66). An aspirate from an epidermal cyst contains much debris and numerous keratinized squamous cells, also anucleate squames (Fig. 2.67). Infected epidermal cysts show similar features to those of subareolar abscess but the latter is usually deeper within the breast and situated near the areola.

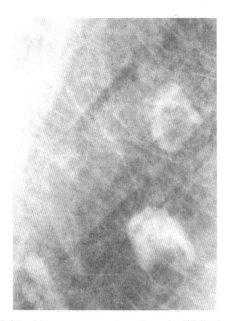

Figure 2.64 Mammogram – lymph node. Whilst lymph nodes are most commonly seen in the axilla or axillary tail region on a mammogram, they can occasionally be seen elsewhere within the breast. Characteristically they have an oval or kidney-shaped appearance. At the hilum of the lymph node there is often fatty replacement which shows up as a low-density area within a more dense oval structure. These two nodules in this illustration show the classical appearance of lymph nodes. Courtesy of Dr Julie Cooke.

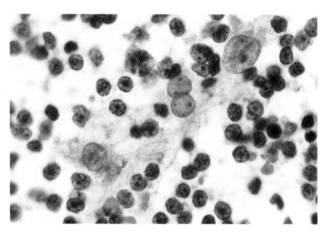

Figure 2.65 Cytology – lymph node. This is an aspirate from an intramammary lymph node showing a mixture of follicle centre cells and small lymphocytes typical of a normal lymph node (Pap).

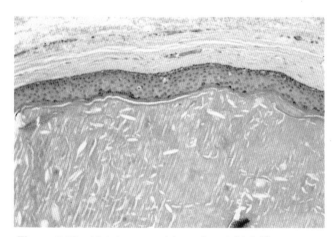

Figure 2.66 Histology – epidermal cyst (H & E).

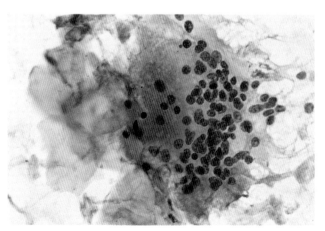

Figure 2.67 Cytology – epidermal cyst. Large multinucleated histiocytes and several anucleate squamous cells are seen. There is no evidence of malignancy (Pap).

REFERENCES

1. Cytology subgroup of the National Coordinating Committee for Breast Cancer Screening Pathology, (eds C. A. Wells, I. O. Ellis, H. D. Zakhour and A. R. Wilson) (1994) Guidelines for cytology procedures and reporting on fine needle aspirates of the breast. *Cytology* **5**, 316–34.

2. Finley, J. L., Silverman, J. F. and Lannin, D. R. (1989) Fine needle aspiration cytology of breast masses in pregnant and lactating women. *Diagn. Cytopathol.* **8**, 255–9.

3. Bloxham, C. A., Shrimauker, J. J., Wadehra, V. and Griffith, C. D. M. (1993) Fine needle aspiration of a lactational focus in a non-pregnant woman. *Cytopathology*, **4**, 243–6.

4. Tavassoli, F. A. and Yeh, I. T. (1987) Lactational and clear cell changes of the breast in non-lactating, non-pregnant women. *Am. J. Clin. Pathol.* **87**, 23–9.

5. Novotny, D. B., Maygarden, S. J., Shermer, R. W. and Frable, W. J. (1991) Fine needle aspiration of benign and malignant breast disease associated with pregnancy. *Acta Cytol.* **35**, 676–86.

6. Grenko, R. T., Lee, K. P. and Lee, K. R. (1990) Fine needle aspiration cytology of lactating ademona of the breast. *Acta Cytol.* **34**, 21–6.

7. Koss, L. G. (1992) *Diagnostic Cytology and its Histopathologic Bases*, 4th edn, J. B. Lippincott Co. Philadelphia. pp. 1299–300.

8. Longacre, T. A. and Bartow, S. A. (1986) A correlative study of human breast and endometrium in the menstrual cycle. *Am. J. Surg. Pathol.* **10**, 382–93.

9. Beller, F. K. and Reiter, R. C. (1990) Benign pathology of the breast. *Current Opinion Obstet. Gynaecol.* **2**, 462–5.

10. Hughes, L. E., Mansel, R. E., Webster, D. J. T. (1987) Aberrations of Normal Development and Involution (ANDI). A new perspective on pathogenesis and nomenclature of benign breast disorder. *Lancet*, **2**, 1316–9.

11. Silverman, J. E., Dabbs, D. J. and Gilbert, C. F. (1983) Fine needle aspiration cytology of adenosis tumour of the breast. *Acta Cytol.* **33**, 181–7.

12. Linnell, F., Ljungberg, O. and Andersson, I. (1980) Breast carcinoma. *Acta Pathol. Microbiol. Scand.* **272**, 14–62.

13. Page, D. L. and Anderson, T. J. (1987) *Diagnostic Histopathology of the Breast*. Churchill Livingstone, Edinburgh, pp. 62–4.

14. Page, D. L. and Anderson, T. J. (1987) *Diagnostic Histopathology of the Breast*. Churchill Livingstone, Edinburgh, pp. 43–50.

15. Ciatto, S., Cariaggi, P. and Bulgaresi, P. (1987) The value of routine cytologic examination of breast cyst fluids. *Acta Cytol.* **31**, 301–4.

16. Nagy, G. K., Jacobs, J. B., Mason-Savas, A. *et al.* (1989) Intracytoplasmic eosinophilic inclusion bodies in breast cyst fluids are giant lysosomes. *Acta Cytol.* **33**, 99–103.

17. Tsuchiya, S., Maruyama, Y., Koike, Y. *et al.* (1987) Cytologic characteristics and origin of naked nuclei in breast aspirate smears. *Acta Cytol.* **31**, 285–90.

18. Stanley, M. W., Tani, E. M. and Skoog, L. (1990) Fine needle aspiration of fibroadenomas of the breast with atypia. *Diagn. Cytopathol.* **6**, 375–81.

19. Goldenberg, V. E., Wiegenstein, L. and Mottet, N. K. (1968) Florid breast fibroadenomas in patients taking hormonal oral contraceptives. *Am. J. Clin. Pathol.* **49**, 52–9.

20. Walker, R. A. (1988) Breast myoepithelium – the ignored cell. *J. Pathol.* **156**, 5–6.

21. Layfield, L. J., Glasgow, B. J. and Cramer, H. (1989) Fine needle aspiration in the management of breast masses. *Pathol. Annu.* **24**, (part 2), 23–62.

22. Whitlatch, S. P. and Panke, T. W. (1987) Myoepithelial cells in needle aspirations of two cases of unusual breast lesions: an aid in differential diagnosis. *Diagn. Cytopathol.* **3**, 77–81.

23. Going, J. J., Anderson, T. J., Wilkinson, S. and Chetty, U. (1987) Granulomatous lobular mastitis. *J. Clin. Pathol.* **40**, 535–40.

24. Macansh, S., Greenberg, M., Barraclough, B. and Pacey, F. (1990) Fine needle aspiration cytology of granulomatous mastitis. *Acta Cytol.* **34**, 38–42.

25. Das, D. K., Sodhani, P., Kashyap, V. *et al.* (1992) Inflammatory lesions of the breast: diagnosis by fine needle aspiration. *Cytopathol.* **3**, 281–9.

26. Houn, H. D. and Granger, J. K. (1991) Granulomatous mastitis secondary to histoplasmosis. *Diagn. Cytopathol.* **7**, 282–5.

27. Dodd, L. G., Sneige, N., Reece, G. P. and Fornage, B. (1993) Fine-needle aspiration cytology of silicone granulomas in the augmented breast. *Diagn. Cytopathol.*, **9**, 498–502.

28. Orell, S. R., Sterrett, G. E., Walters, M. N.-L. and Whitaker, D. (1992) *Manual and Atlas of Fine Needle Aspiration Cytology*, 2nd edn, Churchill Livingstone, Edinburgh.

29. Filomena, C. A., Jordan, A. G. and Ehya, H. (1992) Needle aspiration cytology of the irradiated breast. *Diagn. Cytopathol.* **8**, 327–32.

30. Dornfield, J. M., Thompson, S. K. and Shurbaji, M. S. (1992) Radiation-induced changes in the breast: a potential diagnostic pitfall on fine needle aspiration. *Diagn. Cytopathol.* **8**, 79–81.

31. Bonderson, L. (1987) Aspiration cytology of radiation induced changes of normal breast epithelium. *Acta Cytol.* **31**, 309–10.

32. Peterse, J. L., Thunnissen, F. B. J. M. and van Heerde, P. (1989) Fine needle aspiration cytology of radiation-induced changes in non-neoplastic breast lesions. *Acta Cytol.* **33**, 176–80.

33. Pedio, G., Landoff, U. and Zobeli, L. (1988) Irradiated benign cells of the breast; a potential pitfall in fine needle aspiration cytology. *Acta Cytol.* **32**, 127–8.

34. Kowand, L. M., Verhulst, L. A., Copeland, C. M. and Bose, B. (1984) Epidermal cyst of the breast. *Can. Med. Assoc. J.* **131**, 217–9.

35. Shousha, S. and Maddox, A. (1992) Recurrent epidermal cysts of the breast. *Histopathol.* **21**, 299–300.

3. Malignant appearances

Peter A. Trott

CRITERIA OF MALIGNANCY

As in other topics of diagnostic cytopathology there is no one criterion of malignancy for the interpretation of breast cytology specimens using conventional staining techniques. Despite some advances in the identification of immunological markers that might identify a malignant cell there is as yet none that will do so with any worthwhile degree of specificity and sensitivity. The tyrosine kinase oncogene c-*erb*B-2 appears to be amplified only in breast carcinoma [1] and may therefore be specific but it can be demonstrated in only 30 per cent of invasive carcinomas [2], most of which are high grade and therefore readily recognizable in cytological preparations. Furthermore, in histopathological sections not every cell is reactive so that even in carcinomas in which the oncogene is amplified the needle aspirate specimens may be c-*erb*B-2 negative. The problem of interpretation is further compounded because duct carcinoma *in situ* often shows c-*erb*B-2 positivity so that a positive reaction in a needle aspirate specimen may not necessarily indicate invasive carcinoma [3].

Definitions of the criteria of malignancy have been enumerated by several authors. Oertel and Galblum [4] considered the most important criteria are the cellularity of the specimen and nuclear atypia. Kline *et al.* [5] have published a useful table in which the frequency of features is listed in various types of malignant breast tumours stained by the Papanicolaou technique. Cellularity, dyshesion and monomorphism are important although they emphasize that the degree of abnormality varies with carcinoma type. Useful guidelines are listed by Linsk and Franzen [6]. These consist of the presence of single cells having round or irregularly large nuclei and nucleoli which are best seen in Papanicolaou-stained slides. In addition clusters and bipolar nuclei should be absent. Many of these features are listed in the National Health Service Breast Screening Programme 'Guidelines for Cytology' [7].

In Table 3.1 [8] the criteria of malignancy have been divided into those that are 'obvious' and those that are 'less obvious'. This list is an attempt to provide a consensus of criteria gleaned from the literature and the author's personal experience. The 'obvious' criteria are those generally applied to the identification of malignant cells in all cytological samples with perhaps lack of cohesion being particularly applied to breast aspiration specimens. It is important also to emphasize nuclear border irregularity as this feature occasionally is the only one that tips the balance towards a malignant diagnosis.

The 'less obvious' criteria are worth examining in

Table 3.1   Criteria of malignancy

Obvious	Large size
	Nuclear border irregularity
	Large nucleoli
	Lack of cohesion
	Cellular pleomorphism
Less obvious	Intranuclear vacuoles
	Monomorphism
	Mitoses
	Single cells with much cytoplasm
	Absence of 'benign pairs'

detail. Intranuclear vacuoles may be the counterpart of the intracellular lumina that can be identified by electron microscopy in carcinoma cells [9]. In some cases this may be an important observation in the diagnosis of malignancy although it is certainly also seen in benign specimens. They are seen far more easily in the Giemsa than in the wet-fixed Papanicolaou-stained preparations and are identified as punched-out clear areas about the size of a red blood cell or smaller (Fig. 3.1).

Monomorphism (Fig. 3.2) refers to the type of cell rather than to the degree of variability when comparing one cell with another, and in a smear that is suspicious of malignancy the identification of two

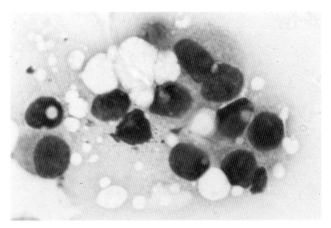

Figure 3.1   High-power view of a cluster of breast carcinoma cells stained with MGG. Many nuclei show vacuoles of various kinds. The one to the left is 'punched out', others less defined.

types of cells, duct epithelial and myoepithelial indicates benignity. In a smear where the cells are all the same type, despite their regularity and sometimes small size, a diagnosis of carcinoma should be considered, although carcinoma is more easily identified when the monomorphic cells show individual pleomorphism.

Mitoses (Fig. 3.3) are seen infrequently in aspirates from carcinomas. This is curious because they are common in histological sections of carcinomas and indeed their presence is an important factor when assessing the histological grade of the tumour

[10]. Their absence in needle aspirates may be the consequence of the comparatively few number of cells present, but the cells are certainly fresh when smeared and it would be unlikely that mitotic activity would complete after the sample has been taken. Nevertheless, their presence is a strong indicator of malignancy although they are known to occur in some benign lesions, notably fibroadenomas.

The observation of single cells with much cytoplasm (Fig. 3.4) has been identified by Linsk and Franzen [6] as a criterion and it is a feature quite

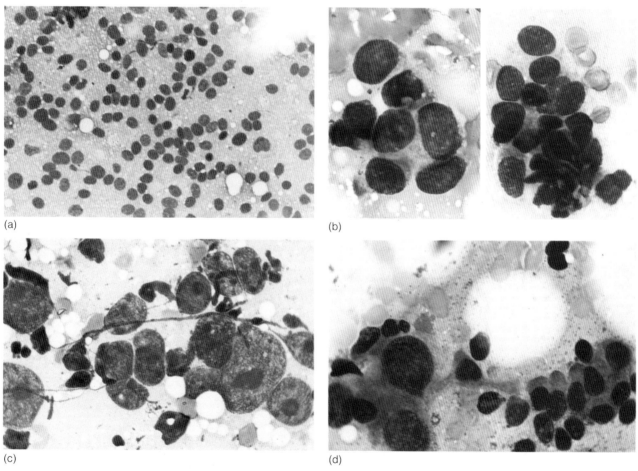

(a)

(b)

(c)

(d)

Figure 3.2 (a) In this low-power photomicrograph the cells are evenly spread and all one type, although they vary in size. This is monomorphism. (b) A high-power photograph showing a cluster of carcinoma cells on the left and cells from a fibroadenoma on the right. Although the carcinoma cells are only slightly larger with irregularity of the nuclear membrane and variation in size, the nuclear consistency is the same. In the cells on the right two types of nuclei can be identified. Some are large and stained palely and others are small with darker nuclei. The cells with the larger nuclei are cuboidal epithelial cells and the smaller ones are myoepithelial. (c) A high-power photomicrograph of cells from a poorly differentiated carcinoma which are extremely pleomorphic, but still show monomorphism. The chromatin staining and the appearance of the nucleoli is similar in each cell. (d) A cluster of benign cells from a proliferative lesion. Two populations of cells can be seen; the smaller are myoepithelial cells and the larger cuboidal epithelial cells.

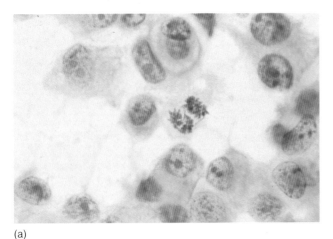

(a)

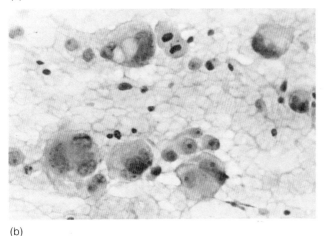

(b)

often found in malignant aspirates. Their presence should raise the alarm that the smear may be malignant and other criteria hunted for enthusiastically.

The absence of 'benign pairs' is a complementary observation to monomorphism as it is a curious fact that myoepithelial cells commonly group together in pairs (Fig. 3.5), and sometimes in clusters of three or even four nuclei (Fig. 3.6). Zajicek [11] recognized single 'sentinel' nuclei and claimed them to be of myoepithelial origin, and maintained that they are very rarely observed in aspirates from carcinoma. Pairs of myoepithelial nuclei which are simply two adjacent sentinel cells, are more easily identified

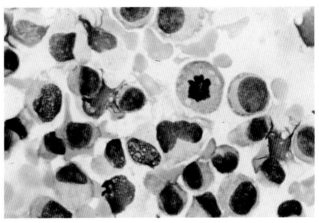

(c)

Figure 3.3 (a) High-power field of a metaphase mitosis stained by the Papanicolaou technique. (b) Low-power field showing a mitosis in a lactational carcinoma stained by Papanicolaou. (c) Prophase mitosis in a cell prepared by the cytospin technique.

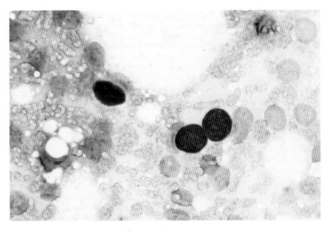

Figure 3.4 Single cells with much cytoplasm, best seen in the lower part of the photomicrograph. When seen singly these cells are a good indicator of malignancy.

Figure 3.5 High-power oil immersion view of a 'pair' of myoepithelial cell nuclei. A single similar nucleus is also present. Note the size in relation to the red blood cells and the consistency of the chromatin.

than single nuclei. Because of their easy identification it is a convenient 'rule of thumb' when confronted with an equivocal smear to hunt for benign pairs of myoepithelial cells and only permit a diagnosis of carcinoma when these are either absent or the atypical cells themselves are large, pleomorphic and irregular, i.e. frankly carcinoma. Observance of this rule will prevent the diagnosis of carcinoma in a fibroadenoma, which often contains large atypical duct epithelial cells, some of which may even be in mitosis, but in which myoepithelial cells singly and in pairs are abundant.

CYTOLOGICAL GRADING

Following the establishment and recognition that histopathological grading has prognostic value [10] and indeed is reproducible, attempts have been made to grade breast carcinoma in needle aspirates. The histopathological factors include the degree of tubule formation, cellular pleomorphism and mitotic rate, the last two being applicable to cytological material. In practice however, as has been stated, mitotic figures are unusual in needle aspirate specimens. However, as a consequence of less traumatic preparative techniques in cytological specimens the increased nuclear detail (particularly in Papanicolaou-stained slides), allows a range of criteria to be assessed and scored according to their

degree of prominence. These include cell dissociation, cell size, cell uniformity, nucleoli, nuclear margin and chromatin patterns.

Although the technology is available for sophisticated analysis and compilation of parameters by automatic image analysis (see Chapter 9), the expense and the time involved in this procedure puts it at a disadvantage. The pathologist requires a grading scheme that can be undertaken on routinely stained material prepared in a conventional manner that is not time consuming. Zajdela et al. [12] related prognosis to the nuclear diameter of aspirated breast cancer cells measured against red blood cells and they reported correlation with histopathological grading and prognosis. This method was expanded by Hunt et al. [13] using more parameters and in Guildford, Robinson et al. [14] established three cytological grades in an analysis of 281 invasive ductal carcinomas which matched well with conventional histological grading.

The advent of neoadjuvant treatment in which carcinomas are treated with chemo- or endocrine therapy after diagnosis by aspiration cytology has highlighted the need for a reliable cytological method of grading. These classification systems are in their infancy but are bound to become more relevant as neoadjuvant treatment becomes consolidated for certain types of tumour, and in which the histological grading, size of tumour and lymph node status are unknown.

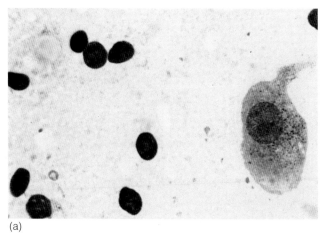

(a)

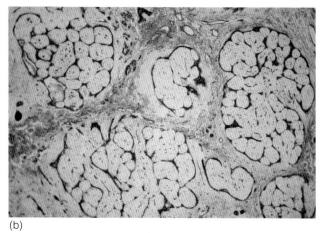

(b)

Figure 3.6 (a) Myoepithelial cell nuclei singly and in triplets. A large normal cuboidal epithelial cell is also present. Aspirate from a fibroadenoma. (b) Fibroadenoma from which the cells in Fig. 6a were aspirated.

BREAST CARCINOMA CLASSIFICATION

Although the main difficulty (and purpose) in breast cytodiagnosis is differentiating benignity from malignancy it is nevertheless appropriate to attempt to match the cytological appearances to the established histopathological classification of breast carcinoma (see Table 3.2) [15]. **Infiltrating duct carcinoma** which comprises nearly 80 per cent of mammary carcinoma, is conveniently divided into those cases **without special features or not otherwise specified (NOS)**, which are the great majority and those **with special features**. Apart from the **rare varieties of**

mammary carcinoma (some of which can be identified on aspiration cytodiagnosis) the next main group of tumours is **infiltrating lobular carcinoma** which provides its own problems for cytological interpretation.

However, it is not the purpose of this book to describe the various histological sub-types of breast carcinoma; it is simply convenient for descriptive purposes to attempt to sub-classify breast carcinoma into the types familiar to surgical pathologists although this is often not possible. Moreover, although the term ductal carcinoma implies that the tumour originates from the breast ducts as opposed

---

Table 3.2 Classification of mammary carcinoma

Tumour type	Approximate % of different types
In situ carcinoma	
In situ duct carcinoma	
(with or without Paget's disease of the nipple; including intracystic carcinoma)	5
In situ lobular carcinoma	3
Infiltrating carcinoma	
Infiltrating duct carcinoma	72
Without special features or not otherwise specified (NOS)	
(with prominent desmoplasia (scirrhous pattern) or without prominent desmoplasia; with or without prominent intraduct carcinoma; with or without Paget's disease of the nipple)	
With special features	
Medullary carcinoma with lymphoid stroma	3
Mucoid carcinoma	2
Tubular carcinoma	2
Infiltrating lobular carcinoma	12
Rare varieties of mammary carcinoma	
Carcinoid tumour of breast	
Signet-ring cell carcinoma	
Secretory or juvenile carcinoma	
Adenoid cystic carcinoma	
Squamous cell carcinoma	
Spindle cell (pseudosarcomatous) carcinoma	
Carcinoma with cartilaginous or osseous metaplasia	
Apocrine carcinoma	
Carcinomas with particular clinical manifestations	
Paget's disease of the nipple	
Inflammatory carcinoma	

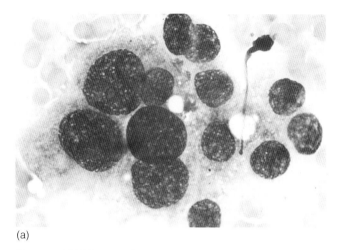

(a)

to lobular carcinoma which is supposed to arise in the lobules, there is no biological proof for this and the distinction is largely concerned with differences in cytological appearances and natural history.

INFILTRATING DUCTAL CARCINOMA (NOS)

Although there is a wide range of appearances, aspirates from infiltrating ductal carcinomas are composed usually of cells that are large and polygonal with a small nuclear cytoplasmic ratio and

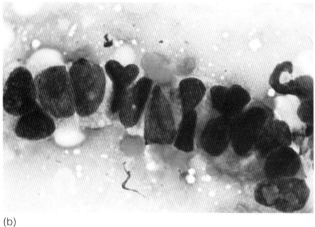

(b)

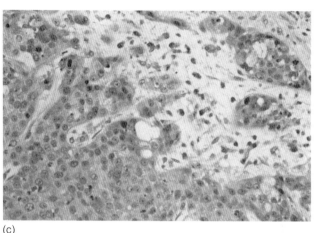

(c)

Figure 3.7 (a) High-power photomicrograph showing large polygonal cells with a small nuclear cytoplasmic ratio. Nucleoli are often multiple and there is marked pleomorphism. To the right of the picture an acinus can be identified. (b) A row of cells showing nuclear moulding, irregular nuclear borders and pleomorphism. (c) Infiltrating poorly differentiated ductal carcinoma.

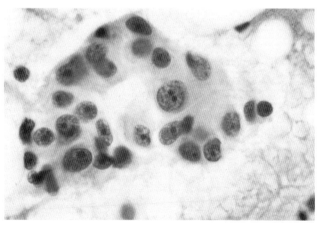

Figure 3.8 High-power view of carcinoma cells stained by Papanicolaou showing prominent nucleoli.

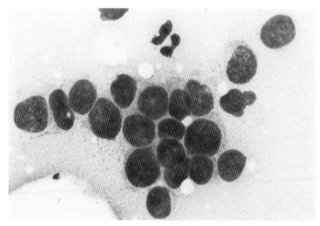

Figure 3.9 Although these cells are small compared to the neutrophil in the upper part of the field they show monomorphism as well as nuclear moulding and some variation in size. These are carcinoma cells from a mass in the upper outer quadrant of the breast in a woman aged 27 years.

marked nuclear border irregularity (Fig. 3.7). In this type of tumour nucleoli are easily identified and often multiple. The Papanicolaou-stained cells show this well (Fig. 3.8). In other tumours the aspirated cells are medium-sized and grouped in loose aggregates in which the monomorphic appearance of the nuclei is striking (Fig. 3.9). It is these tumours that will often have single cells within the smear that are recognized as being abnormal according to the criteria of malignancy.

In many cases, particularly high grade tumours, the diagnosis of carcinoma is straightforward and the aspirate reveals loose sheets and single large pleomorphic irregular cells conforming to the 'obvious' criteria of malignancy (Table 3.1) that are quickly recognized as adenocarcinoma. Occasional blobs of intracellular mucin (Fig. 3.10) are seen as well as cells containing cytoplasmic granules which may indicate neuroendocrine differentiation (Fig. 3.11). Sometimes the finding of granules may confirm suspicions of malignancy and allow a positive diagnosis to be made.

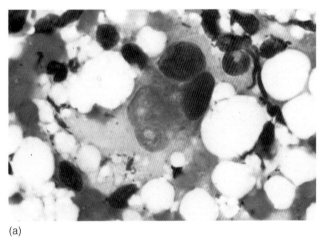

(a)

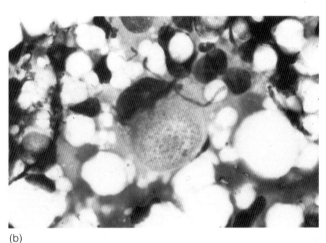

(b)

Figure 3.10 (a) High-power view of a carcinoma cell showing pink staining mucin in the cytoplasm. (b) Another cell from the same patient also showing intracellular mucin.

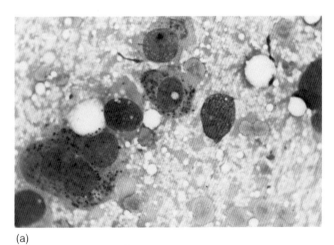

(a)

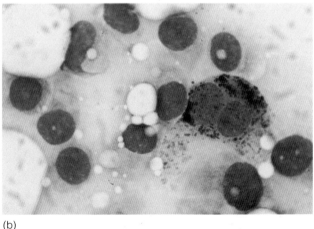

(b)

Figure 3.11 (a) Many cells show basophilic granules in the cytoplasm. These are certainly epithelial cells and these granules probably indicate neuroendocrine differentiation. This is common in breast cancer and in aspiration cytology of the breast, their presence may help in establishing a diagnosis of carcinoma. (b) A binucleate cell has numerous granules in its cytoplasm which are spilling out through the fractured plasma membrane. Note that the other cells are devoid of granules.

LOBULAR CARCINOMA

Infiltrating lobular carcinoma comprises 12 per cent of cases of mammary carcinoma (see Table 3.2). It has a characteristic histological appearance which includes the classic appearances and three variants, solid, alveolar, and mixed [16]. It is more often bilateral than ductal carcinoma and is thought to spread selectively to liver and abdominal organs.

Antoniades and Spector [17] studied nine cases of lobular carcinoma in which they examined imprints which were compared with histological sections both thick and thin. A range of cell sizes was seen, from those just larger than a lymphocyte with a small round to oval nucleus, to signet ring forms with a nuclear size up to 11.8 micrometres and big cytoplasmic vacuoles containing mucin (Fig. 3.12). The typical cell was a small one with a round-to-oval nucleus and finely dispersed chromatin with a small distinct nucleolus and cytoplasm with punched-out vacuoles. Leach and Howell [18] also examined nine cases and found that in needle aspirates the classic variety was the most likely to result in a false negative cytodiagnosis. The importance of cytoplasmic vacuoles is again emphasized. However, a few cases of the alveolar variant had large cells and were misdiagnosed as ductal carcinoma.

Two kinds of cells have been generally described in aspirates from lobular carcinoma. Firstly, loosely dispersed sheets of small cells seen particularly in postmenopausal women and secondly, tight clusters of pleomorphic cells seen in three-dimensional groups. The small cells are often only slightly larger than red blood cells and can be mistaken for an intramammary lymph node or even malignant lymphoma (Fig. 3.13). The diagnosis is often suspected on low-power microscopy when diffuse sheets of cells are seen and a prolonged hunt at high power usually reveals one or two cells with quite a lot of cytoplasm and others in which epithelial clustering is apparent. This pattern was recognized by Zajicek [11] and called 'carcinoma, small cell type'. Experience is required to identify these cases.

Those cases that present in aspirates with clusters can also be difficult to recognize. There is however, usually nuclear moulding as well as irregular nuclear

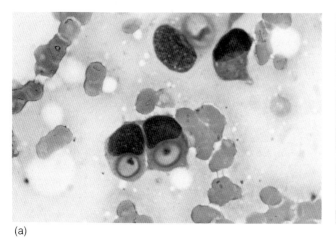

(a)

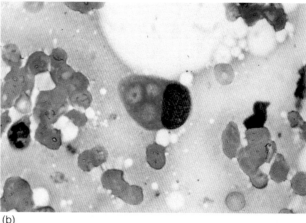

(b)

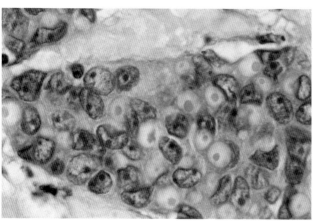

(c)

Figure 3.12 (a) Two cells are seen centrally with vacuoles in their cytoplasm in which a small blob of mucus is present. These appearances have been described in aspirates from infiltrating lobular carcinoma although (as in this case) the histological appearances were more in favour of a ductal lesion. (b) Here a cell shows three vacuoles each of which contains mucus. (c) High-power photomicrograph of the histopathology section of the case shown in (a) and (b). Note the blobs of mucin in the cytoplasmic vacuoles. These are PAS positive.

outlines towards the periphery of the cluster and in these smears there may also be loose groups of rather larger irregular cells that support the diagnosis but these may be few and far between.

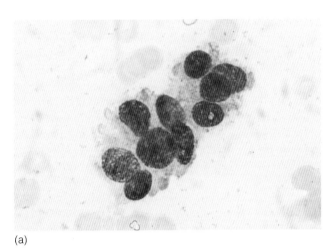

(a)

Figure 3.13 (a) Cells aspirated from a classical infiltrating lobular carcinoma. Note the small size of the nuclei compared to the red blood cells. The true nature of this lesion can be difficult to assess in an aspirate. Examination

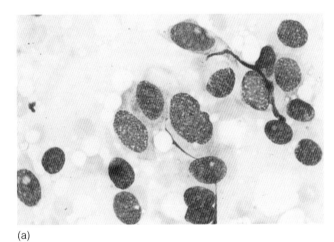

(a)

Figure 3.14 (a) These cells were aspirated from a patient with duct carcinoma *in situ*. The cells are certainly malignant on account of the irregularity of the nuclear border, their pleomorphism and increased size. It is not possible to differentiate this lesion from an infiltrating carcinoma. (b) Another field showing the dyshesion of the cells which are also monomorphic. (c) Histological section of duct carcinoma *in situ* from the case aspirated and illustrated in (a) and (b).

IN SITU CARCINOMA

Although there have been reports of the characteristic appearances of cells aspirated from purely *in situ*

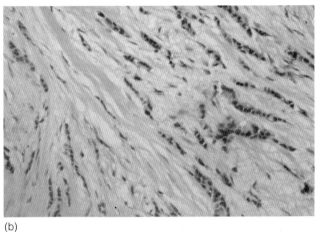

(b)

under oil immersion can be helpful. (b) Histological section of the same case as in (a) showing the linear infiltration of lobular carcinoma.

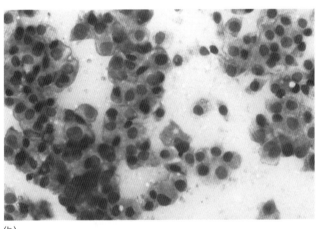

(b)

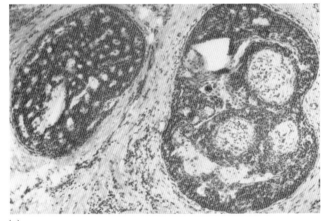

(c)

lesions [19] there is no single criterion that will differentiate this lesion from aspirates of infiltrating carcinomas. The diagnosis is a histopathological one and depends on the characteristic appearances that diagnose duct carcinoma *in situ* with its variants or lobular carcinoma *in situ* which is found incidentally when biopsies are undertaken for benign disease. In the latter lesion, the cells are small and round but in ductal carcinoma *in situ* they are often very large and contain prominent nucleoli (Fig. 3.14).

It may be possible with the aid of the mammographic diagnosis showing characteristic microcalcification to conclude that individual lesions are most likely ductal carcinoma *in situ* rather than invasive carcinoma. However, the cytopathological criteria are too imprecise to indicate this diagnosis in every example.

MEDULLARY CARCINOMA

These lesions are circumscribed carcinomas [20] composed of structureless sheets of large pleomorphic cells, sometimes with bizarre-shaped nuclei with a marked lymphoid stroma in which plasma cells and lymphocytes are numerous. They occur at all ages and have a better prognosis than the high degree of epithelial atypia would predict. However, focal small areas of lymphoid stroma are quite common in high grade ductal carcinoma and the diagnosis of medullary carcinoma must be reserved for those in which the lymphoid component is at least 90 per cent of the tumour bulk.

Needle aspirates from such lesions show these features very clearly (Fig. 3.15). The cells are very large and have prominent nucleoli and are disaggregated. The lymphoid stroma is easily identified and plasma cells are numerous. However, it is not possible in every case to be certain that within the bulk of the lesion a large proportion will show evidence of conventional ductal carcinoma and so not conform to the strict histopathological criteria. Nevertheless, it is possible to suggest to the clinicians that this may be a medullary carcinoma particularly when the characteristic mammographic appearances of a circumscribed nodule are also seen.

It has been the author's and other's experience [21] that some medullary carcinomas produce cystic

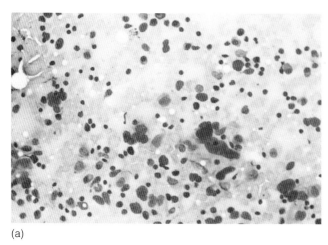

(a)

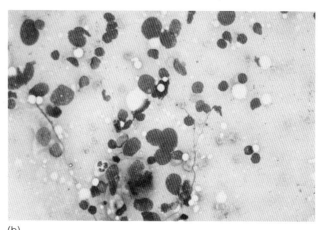

(b)

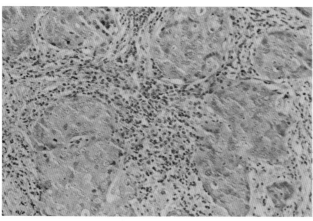

(c)

Figure 3.15 (a) Low-power photomicrograph showing several clusters of very large irregular cells with a background of inflammatory cells. Many of these are plasma cells and lymphocytes. (b) Large irregular carcinoma cells are present as well as inflammatory cells. (c) The characteristic histopathological appearances of medullary carcinoma.

fluid when aspirated. In three cases of this kind the fluid has been up to 2 cm in volume and only slightly bloodstained. The cells in this example were large and pleomorphic and the lymphoid stroma abundant.

MUCOID (MUCINOUS) CARCINOMA

In this lesion the carcinoma clusters are surrounded by extracellular mucin. The appearances are very characteristic on needle aspiration cytodiagnosis [22] especially in Giemsa preparations. The mucus appears in pink or purple bands throughout the smear and the carcinoma cells often appear lined up alongside the mucus (Fig. 3.16). The cells themselves are usually quite small and not pleomorphic. The diagnosis may be difficult when the mucus is either scanty or badly stained and as the cells are small and relatively monomorphic the diagnosis may be overlooked.

Stanley *et al.* [23] investigated the cytological appearances of pure mucinous carcinoma and mixed infiltrating ductal and mucinous carcinoma. They identified features indicative of pure mucinous carcinoma consisting of abundant mucin in all smears, no pleomorphism and no necrosis. It is important if possible to identify mucinous carcinoma as those cases conforming to the histopathological criteria (i.e. at least 90 per cent of the tumour being mucinous) have a good prognosis [24].

PAPILLARY CARCINOMA

Histologically these tumours are circumscribed lesions occurring in any part of the breast but most notably beneath the nipple usually in post-menopausal women. The distinction must be made between invasive and non-invasive papillary carcinoma, the latter having the worse prognosis. Papillary carcinoma is composed of branching fronds covered by stratified atypical epithelium appearing similar to that seen in ductal carcinoma *in situ*, and indeed cribriform and solid areas may be present.

Needle aspirates are often cystic and blood-contaminated. The cells are usually less pleomorphic than in carcinoma NOS and may be in papillary clusters (Fig. 3.17). Myoepithelial cells, forming pairs of nuclei are absent. In practice interpretation is usually difficult and an equivocal diagnosis may be the safest. The problem is compounded by the presence of papillary patterns in some examples of complex sclerosing lesions but in aspirates from such lesions a mixture of papillary clusters, benign pairs and single 'naked' nuclei will be seen.

SARCOMA

Malignant mesenchymal tumours of the breast are divided into those with an epithelial component and those without. Those with epithelium are malignant phyllodes tumours and are described in Chapter 5.

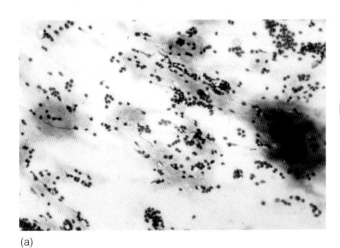

(a)

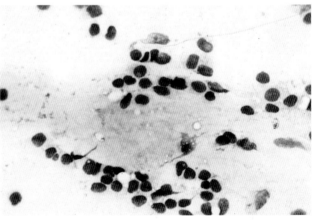

(b)

Figure 3.16 (a) Low-power photomicrograph of a needle aspirate showing the characteristic features of a mucinous carcinoma. Broad streaks of pink-staining mucin are present with loose aggregates and single intervening cells. (b) At high power the cells are small but monomorphic and appear to be lined up along the edge of the mucin. The Giemsa stain is particularly useful in the diagnosis of this type of carcinoma. In the Papanicolaou-stained smears mucin is almost invisible.

Sarcomas without an epithelial component are less common than malignant phyllodes tumours and are usually fibrosarcomas. However, the breast is a site where heterologous elements within a sarcoma are found such as osteoid, cartilage, muscle and fat, and sarcomatous metaplasia is not uncommon in carcinoma. Histopathological specimens of sarcoma are thoroughly sectioned to exclude foci of conventional carcinoma which can be confirmed with appropriate immunohistochemistry.

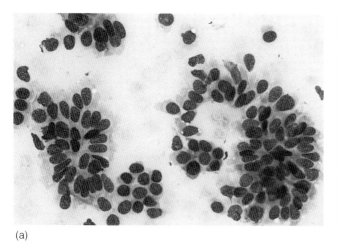

(a)

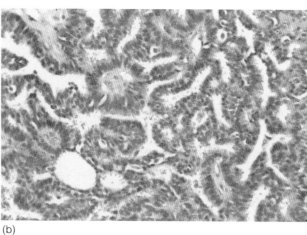

(b)

Figure 3.17 (a) Clusters of monomorphic cells aspirated from a circumscribed lesion in an elderly lady. The groups of cells show a papillary pattern, particularly the clusters to the left of the photomicrograph in which there is nuclear palisading. (b) Counterpart histology showing a papillary carcinoma.

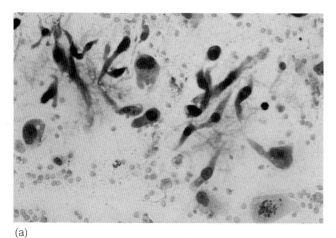

(a)

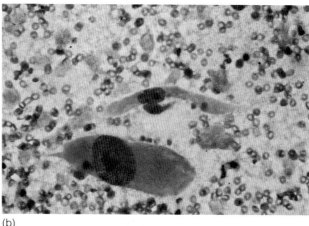

(b)

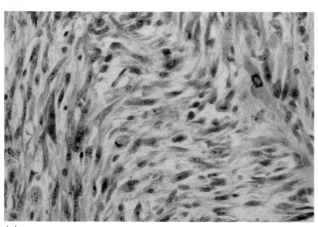

(c)

Figure 3.18 (a) Cells aspirated from a soft lump in the inner quadrant of the breast in a 64-year-old woman. Numerous elongated spindle cells are present. (b) One very large bizarre-shaped cell is seen and another that is elongated. Note that in cytological preparations all the cell is included on the slide rather than a section through it. (c) The histology showed a fibrosarcoma.

Consequently the cytodiagnosis of breast sarcoma is fraught with difficulties and even when good-quality samples containing spindle cells typical of sarcoma seen in other body sites are obtained (Fig. 3.18), the cytodiagnosis of breast sarcoma should be made with circumspection. The only situation where sarcoma can be confidentially diagnosed in a breast needle aspirate is in recurrent sarcoma in which the primary tumour has been properly sampled and assessed histopathologically.

REFERENCES

1. Borresen, A., Ottestad, L., Gaustad, A. *et al.* (1990) Amplification and protein over-expression of the neu/Her-2/c-*erb*B2 protooncogene in human breast carcinomas: relationship to loss of gene sequences on chromosome 17, family history and prognosis. *Br. J. Cancer*, **62**, 585–90.
2. Gusterson, B. A., Machin, L. G., Gullick, W. J. and Wright, C. (1988) c-*erb*B-2 Expression in benign and malignant breast disease. *Br. J. Cancer* **5**, 453–8.
3. Allan, S. M., Fernando, I. N., Sandle, J. and Trott, P. A. (1993) Expression of the c-*erb*B-2 gene product as detected in cytologic aspirates in breast cancer. *Acta Cytol.* **37**, 981–2.
4. Oertel, Y. C. and Galbum, L. L. Fine needle aspiration of the breast; Diagnostic criteria. *Pathol. Annu.*, **18**, 375–407.
5. Kline, T. S., Kannan, V. and Kline, I. K. (1985) Appraisal and cytomorphologic analysis of common carcinomas of the breast. *Diagn. Cytopathol.* **1**, 188–93.
6. Linsk, J. A. and Franzen, S. (1983) *Clinical Aspiration Cytology*, J. B. Lippincott, Philadelphia, pp. 114–5.
7. Cytology subgroup of the National Co-ordinating Committee for Breast Cancer Screening Pathology, (eds. C. A. Wells, I. O. Ellis, H. D. Zakhour and A. R. Wilson) (1994) Guidelines for cytology procedures and reporting on fine needle aspirates of the breast. *Cytology* **5**, 316–34.
8. Trott, P. A. (1991) Aspiration cytodiagnosis of the breast. *Diagn. Oncol.* **1**, 79–87.
9. Fisher, E. R. (1976) Ultrastructure of the human breast and its disorders. *Am. J. Clin. Path.* **66**, 291–375.
10. Elston, C. W. and Ellis, I. O. (1992) Pathological prognostic factors in breast cancer. *Histopathology*, **19**, 403–10.
11. Zajicek, J. (1974) Aspiration biopsy cytology part 1; Cytology of supradiaphragmatic organs in *Monographs in Clinical Cytology*, (ed. G. L. Weid), S. Karger, Basel.
12. Zajdela, A., DeLaRiva, L. and Ghossein, N. (1984) The relation of prognosis to the nuclear diameter of breast cancer cells obtained by cytologic aspirations. *Acta Cytol.* **23**, 75–80.
13. Hunt, C. M., Ellis, I. O., Elston, C. W. *et al.* (1990) Cytological grading of breast carcinoma – a feasible proposition? *Cytopathology*, **1**, 287–95.
14. Robinson, I. A., McKee, G., Nicholson, A. *et al.* (1994) Prognostic value of cytological grading of fine-needle aspirates from breast carcinomas. *Lancet*, **343**, 947–9.
15. Millis, R. (1984) *Atlas of Breast Pathology*, MTP Press Ltd, Lancaster,
16. Page, D. L. and Anderson, T. J. (1987) *Diagnostic Histopathology of the Breast*, Churchill Livingstone, Edinburgh, p. 219.
17. Antoniades, K. and Spector, H. B. (1987) Similarities and variations among lobular carcinoma cells. *Diagn. Cytopathol.* **3**, 55–9.
18. Leach, C. and Howell, L. P. (1992) Cytodiagnosis of classic lobular carcinoma and its variants. *Acta Cytol.* **36**, 199–202.
19. Sneige, N., White, V. A., Katz, R. L. *et al.* Ductal carcinoma-*in-situ* of the breast: fine-needle aspiration cytology of 12 cases.
20. Ridolphi, R. L., Rosen, P. P., Port, A. *et al.* (1977) Medullary carcinoma of the breast; A clinicopathologic study with ten year follow-up. *Cancer*, **40**, 1365–85.
21. Howell, L. P. and Kline, T. S. (1990) Medullary carcinoma of the breast; a rare cytologic finding in cyst fluid aspirates. *Cancer*, **65**, 277–82.
22. Duane, G. B., Canter, M. H., Branigan, T. and Chang, C. (1987) A morphologic and morphometric study of cells from colloid carcinoma of the breast obtained by fine needle aspiration. *Acta Cytol.* **31**, 742–50.
23. Stanley, M. W., Tani, E. M. and Skoog, L. (1989) Mucinous breast carcinoma and mixed mucinous infiltrating ductal carcinoma: A comparative cytologic study. *Diagn. Cytopathol.* **5**, 134–8.
24. Clayton, F. (1986) Pure mucinous carcinomas of breast; Morphologic features and prognostic correlates. *Human Path.* **17**, 34–8.

4. Equivocal appearances

Peter A. Trott

INTRODUCTION

In this chapter a number of cases are presented and illustrated in which the cytological appearances of the breast needle aspirate has been equivocal or 'suspicious'. In Chapter 1 the diagnostic classifications of C1, C2, C3, C4 and C5 are explained and in this section cases classified as C3 (atypia probably benign) and C4 (suspicious of malignancy) are illustrated and the lessons to be learnt detailed.

To the trained surgical histopathologist but novice cytopathologist, about two-thirds of needle aspirates from carcinoma cases will be obvious carcinoma provided they are good quality specimens. The experienced diagnostic cytopathologist who takes his own needle aspirates will diagnose carcinoma in well over 90 per cent of cases. Therefore, depending on training and experience, there will always be cases that present diagnostic difficulties and remain equivocal in their interpretation. The following case histories will highlight these problems.

Compared to cervical cytopathology there are no grades of epithelial abnormality that relate to a state of precancerous or intra-epithelial neoplasia. All breast lumps are either benign or malignant with a few exceptions that exercise the minds of very experienced breast histopathologists. In cytologically equivocal cases it is sound practice to proceed to the next diagnostic test, whether this be Tru-cut core biopsy or surgical incision or excision, and the cytopathologist should not expect that all cases can be definitively diagnosed. In the Guidelines for Breast Cytology Screening it is stated that 'a C5 malignant diagnosis is one in which the interpreter should feel at ease in making such a diagnosis' [1]. When the interpreter is not at ease for whatever reason the diagnosis will be equivocal.

Cases 1 to 6 have been illustrated by paintings as well as conventional photomicrography. These paintings were undertaken by a skilled medical artist, Mr Peter Walsh of the Medical Art Department of the Royal Marsden Hospital, of fields selected by the author in order to illustrate specific features [2]. The purpose of this is to provide an alternative teaching medium to photomicrography and thereby avoid artefacts that are inherent in the photographic technique. Peter Walsh sat at the microscope and painted the cells directly as he saw them so that they are therefore his artistic interpretation.

The work of trained medical artists has become less fashionable since the technological advances of photomicrography but in former years they provided illustrations for many famous cytopathology text books, e.g. Dr Papanicolaou's *Atlas of Exfoliative Cytology* [3] and the first edition of Dr Sprigg's book on serous effusions [4]. It was thought that paintings of this kind might provide additional information for those learning to interpret breast aspiration cytopathology as an alternative to photomicrographs.

CASE 1

Painting 1 is an aspirate from a 4 cm lump in the left breast in a lady aged 73 years. The sample was a cellular one which consisted of loose clusters and single monomorphic cells showing slight enlargement and little chromatin abnormality or nucleolar enlargement. The interpretation was difficult but in view of the lady's age the cells were thought probably to be carcinoma. The report issued was 'suspicious of carcinoma, C4'.

The painting can be compared with the high-power photomicrograph (Fig. 4.1a). In the painting the red blood cells are more clearly illustrated and a lymphocyte has been 'brought in' from an adjacent field in order to compare the size of the epithelial nuclei. The nuclei are of similar size with very little border irregularity and a diffuse chromatin pattern. From the morphological point of view, the loose association and the absence of a double population of epithelial cells support a diagnosis of carcinoma. However, the cytological appearances are not abnormal enough to warrant a certain diagnosis of malignancy.

Figure 4.1b is a low-power view illustrating the loose appearance of the cell clusters. In Fig. 4.1c there is a suggestion of a double population of epithelial cells. At the top right-hand corner the nuclei are enlarged and look very atypical, but smaller cells are also present, some of which have pyknotic nuclei that may well be myoepithelial in origin. An epithelial cluster with an adjacent polymorph to show the small size of the nuclei is present in Fig. 4.1d. Figure 4.1e shows the low-power appearance of the histology of the excised specimen. Acinar clusters are seen with monomorphic cells indicating a grade 1, well-differentiated infiltrating ductal carcinoma. Figure 4.1f is a high-power photomicrograph of the histopathology slide. Here, the monomorphic appearance of the individual nuclei is well seen for comparison with the cytology.

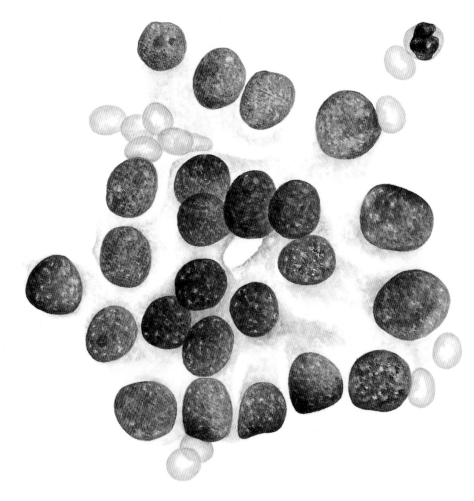

Painting 1

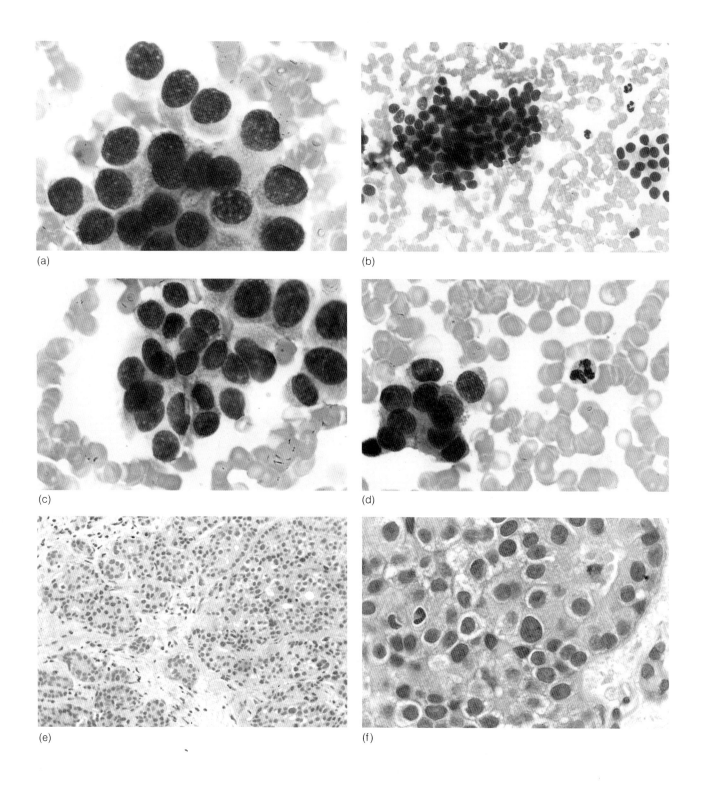

(a)

(b)

(c)

(d)

(e)

(f)

CASE 2

The cells illustrated in Painting 2 were aspirated from a 1.5 cm mass in the upper outer quadrant of the right breast from a 46-year-old woman. Clinically the mass was mobile and was thought to be a fibroadenoma. This diagnosis was supported by the ultrasound examination which indicated a solid lesion.

The cells in Fig. 4.2a can be compared with the painting in which there is a well-defined cluster of epithelial cells showing moderate enlargement and some variation in size and shape. Although there is some moulding of the nuclei it is possible to differentiate most nuclei into one or another type. In the centre of the field there are smaller darker nuclei that are probably myoepithelial in origin.

Despite this, and taking into account the patient's age the report indicated that these cells were 'atyp-ical, C3'. Excision biopsy was undertaken and a fibroadenoma diagnosed histologically.

In Fig. 4.2b, crush artefact has artificially increased the atypical appearances with a suggestion of an intracytoplasmic vacuole in the centre of the field. At the bottom left-hand corner a well-preserved myoepithelial cell nucleus is present. The cells in Fig. 4.2c look crowded and show pleomorphism. No certain evidence of myoepithelial nuclei is present. The low-power photomicrograph (Fig. 4.2d) is of an intracanalicular fibroadenoma, and Fig. 4.2e shows a high-power photomicrograph of an epithelial cleft taken at the same magnification as the cytology. In the latter, the atypical appearances of the epithelial cells can be seen. Some of the cells have prominent nucleoli and others are elongated. Scattered myoepithelial nuclei are also seen.

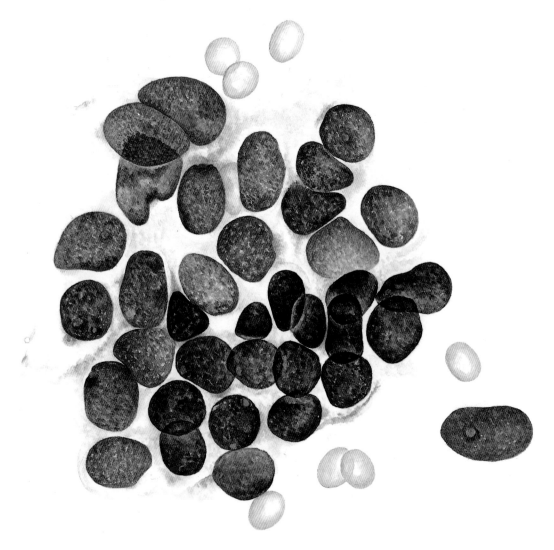

Painting 2

54

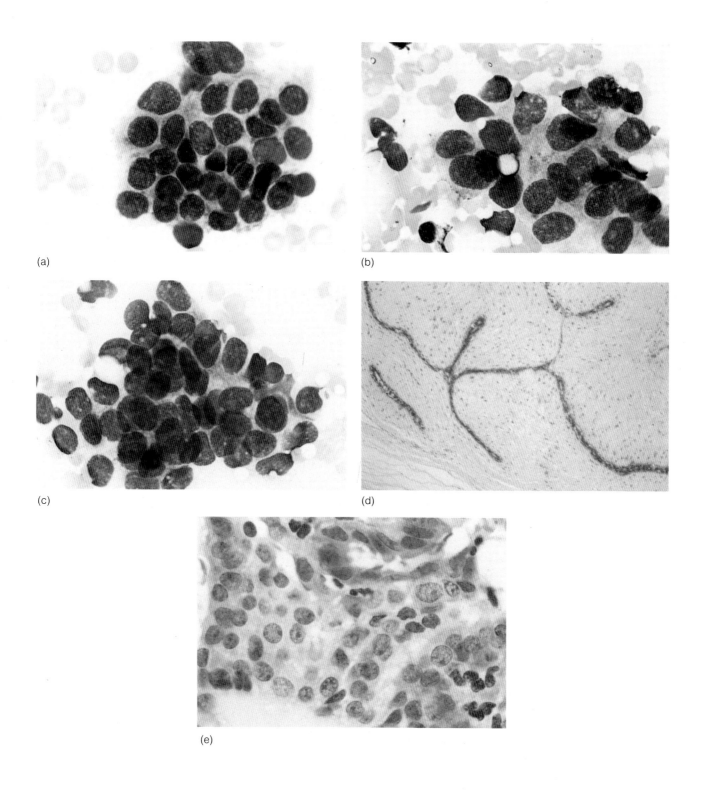

(a)

(b)

(c)

(d)

(e)

CASE 3

Painting 3 is an aspirate from an area of nodularity above the left nipple in a lady aged 61 years. No specific mass was felt but there was a positive family history and the mammographic appearances were atypical.

The aspirate consisted of loose aggregates of monomorphic cells showing variations in size and shape and prominent intranuclear vacuoles. The nuclear chromatin was diffuse and the nucleoli were not prominent. The cells in the painting can be compared with those in the photomicrograph (Fig. 4.3a). In the centre of the field there is a suggestion of cytoplasmic granularity. This specimen was dif-

ficult to interpret. The report was issued 'suspicious of carcinoma, C4'.

Figure 4.3b shows the loose sheets of pleomorphic cells. Several pairs of nuclei that resemble myoepithelial cells are seen in Fig. 4.3c. These features are an indication of benignity and when found with atypical cells there must be no doubt that the atypical cells are 'malignant' before a positive diagnosis of carcinoma can be issued. In this case although atypical, the abnormal cells could not be designated certainly malignant. Figure 4.3d shows a well-differentiated infiltrating ductal carcinoma and Fig. 4.3e is carcinoma surrounding a benign duct.

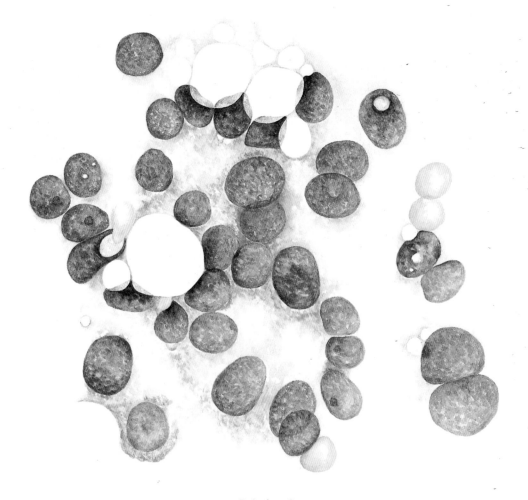

Painting 3

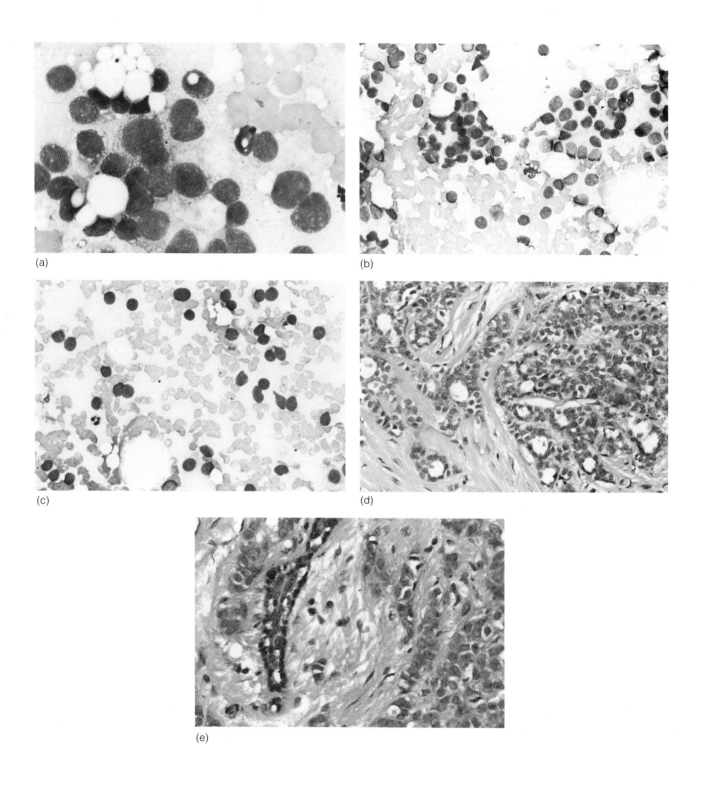

(a)

(b)

(c)

(d)

(e)

CASE 4

The cells in Painting 4 were aspirated from a small lump in the left breast of a 37-year-old woman. The sample was a cellular one showing some atypical features. Clinically, the mass was thought to be benign and the mammogram showed no significant abnormality.

The cells in the painting and the photomicrograph (Fig. 4.4a) show considerable variation in shape and there are intranuclear vacuoles present. Despite this the borders of the cluster are fairly regular and in the bottom centre a rather squashed cell with a darker nucleus is present that may well be a myoepithelial nucleus. The smears were reported as 'atypical appearances, C3'. After a year the lump was no longer palpable and the patient was discharged.

In this high-power field (Fig. 4.4b) there is variation in nuclear size but the chromatin appears finally dispersed. Careful observation will reveal several cells that are probably myoepithelial in origin. Many nuclei are elongated and there is definite irregularity of the nuclear border in Fig. 4.4c. Some of these appearances may be artefactual.

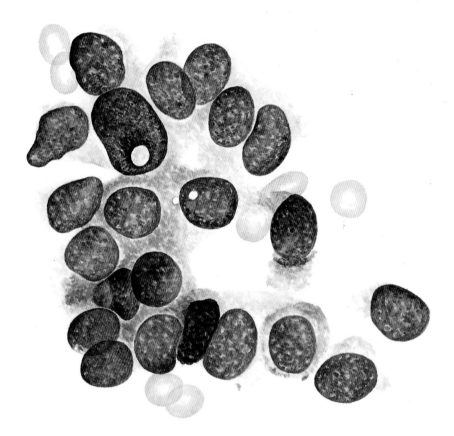

Painting 4

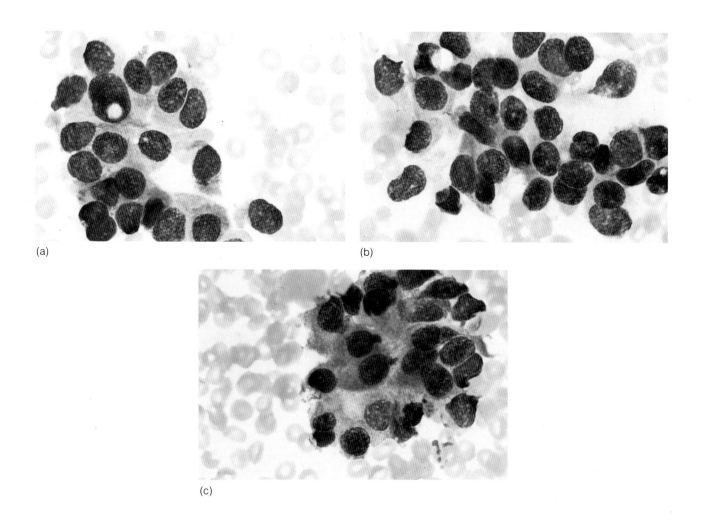

(a)

(b)

(c)

CASE 5

Painting 5 is an aspirate from a mass in the lower inner quadrant of the right breast in a woman aged 69 years. The mass measured 1.5 cm in diameter and although hard on palpation was not fixed.

A good-quality smear was obtained which showed the atypical groups of epithelial cells illustrated in Fig. 4.5a and the painting. The nuclei vary considerably in size but have a generally round shape with little nuclear border irregularity. However, no myoepithelial nucleus is present in the cluster and the cells are generally monomorphic. Although suspicious of malignancy they were considered not atypical enough to provide a categoric diagnosis. This sample was reported 'cells highly suspicious of malignancy C4'.

In Fig. 4.5b some central cells perhaps appear different to others. These suggest the presence of myoepithelial cell nuclei. Generally, the cells in this group show atypical features with nuclear moulding and variation in size. Figure 4.5c shows cells scattered within the cluster that could be myoepithelial nuclei. The larger nuclei are round or oval in shape with little atypia. The cells in Fig. 4.5d are bunched together to form a syncytium. Little atypia is present. A wide local excision and axillary dissection (Fig. 4.5e) was performed which revealed a poorly differentiated grade 3 infiltrating ductal carcinoma composed of broad bands of atypical cells in which nucleoli and nuclear pleomorphism were prominent. Figure 4.5f is a high-power photomicrograph taken at the same magnification as the cytology pictures. Although visible, the nucleoli are not particularly large and indeed there are smaller nuclei scattered throughout that were also seen in the aspirate specimen and thought to be myoepithelial nuclei.

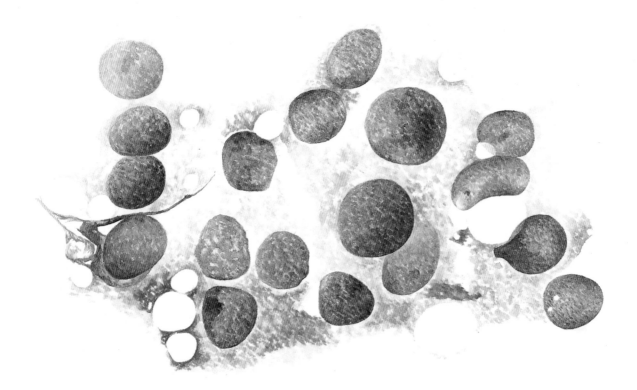

Painting 5

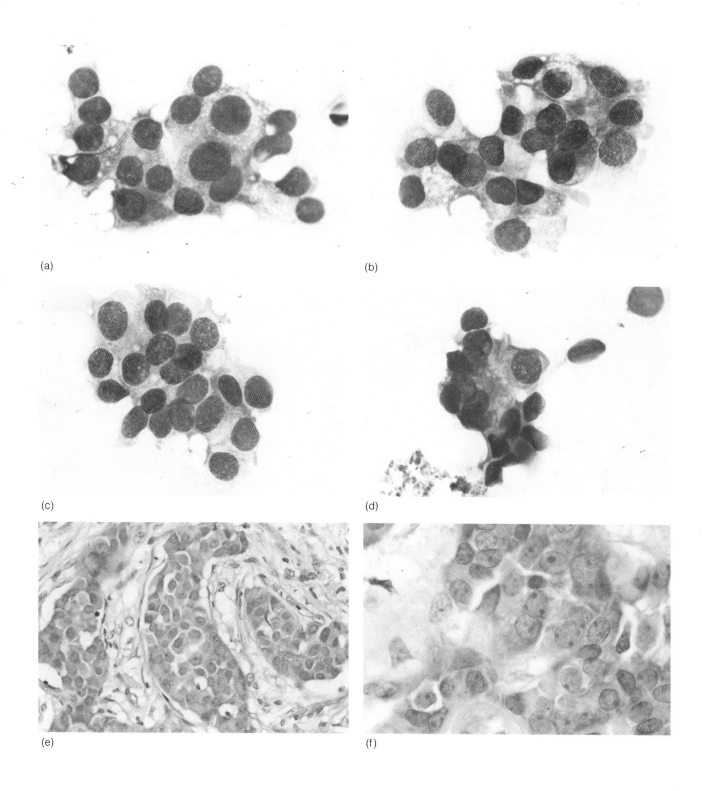

(a)

(b)

(c)

(d)

(e)

(f)

CASE 6

The cells in Painting 6 were aspirated from a small mass in the right breast of a woman aged 45 years. Mammographically and at ultrasound a solid lesion compatible with a fibroadenoma was evident. The photomicrograph (Fig. 4.6a) of the same field as the painting shows monomorphic cells with dispersed chromatin and only little nuclear border irregularity. In the painting a 'pair' of myoepithelial nuclei have been 'brought in'. These were situated outside the relevant field (see Fig. 4.6b) and provided the clue to the diagnosis. Despite this however, the nuclei were abnormal and many atypical. A diagnosis of 'cells with worrying features present, C3'. Six months later the patient reported that the lump had disappeared and two years later she is well and asymptomatic. No operation was performed.

A pair of myoepithelial cells is present on the left of the photomicrograph, Fig. 4.6b. Figure 4.6c shows a cluster of irregular cells showing fragmentation of the border of the cluster and in Fig. 4.6d the cells show rather more organization but many are atypical.

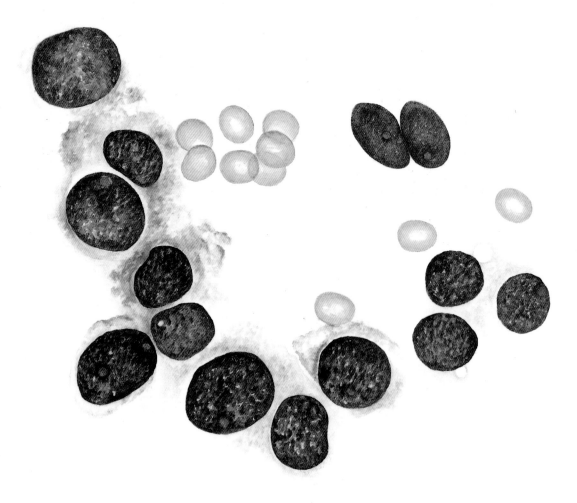

Painting 6

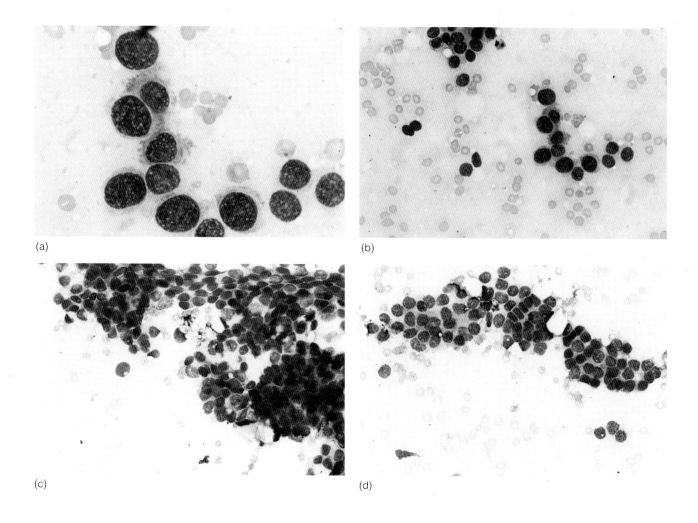

(a)

(b)

(c)

(d)

CASE 7

Case 7 is a nipple smear specimen from a 74-year-old lady with a short history of a blood-stained discharge. On physical examination a mass was also felt below the nipple. Few cells were obtained but some were very atypical. These were reported as 'highly suspicious of malignancy C4'.

In Fig. 4.7a blown-out cells are present with eccentric nuclei and vacuolated cytoplasm. Although the nuclei are indistinct they are extremely large compared to the red blood cells in the background. These cells resemble adenocarcinoma. The cells shown in Fig. 4.7b are more evenly spread but are similarly very large with rather bubbly cytoplasm. Note the increased size of the nuclei compared to the red blood cells in the top left hand corner of the photomicrograph. Figure 4.7c is a photomicrograph of the histology of the underlying mass. This is an intraductal papillary carcinoma showing focal stromal infiltration. Finally, Fig. 4.7d is a high-power photograph of the cells seen in the histology at similar magnification to the cytology specimen. Similar cells are identified.

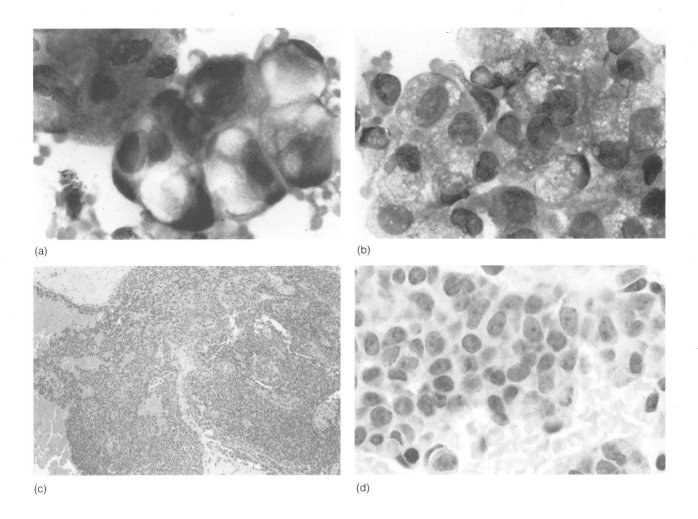

(a)

(b)

(c)

(d)

CASE 8

Case 8 is an aspirate from an area of diffuse thickening in the upper outer quadrant of the breast in a woman aged 57 years.

The cells illustrated in Fig. 4.8a are in loose groups and singly but one tight cluster is present. The striking feature is their small size. Compared to the red blood cells in the background they are not much larger than lymphocytes. Certainly intramammary lymph node and even lymphoma should be considered in the differential diagnosis but the cluster on the right of the photomicrograph is certainly epithe-lial. In Fig. 4.8b a polymorph is present which appears larger than the epithelial cells. The features of this case are very distinctive but their correct interpretation requires experience. The histology (Fig. 4.8c) showed infiltrating lobular carcinoma in which sheets of small pleomorphic carcinoma cells were present as well as others infiltrating stroma. These cases can be called 'small cell carcinoma' and usually they are shown to be infiltrating lobular carcinoma at histological biopsy.

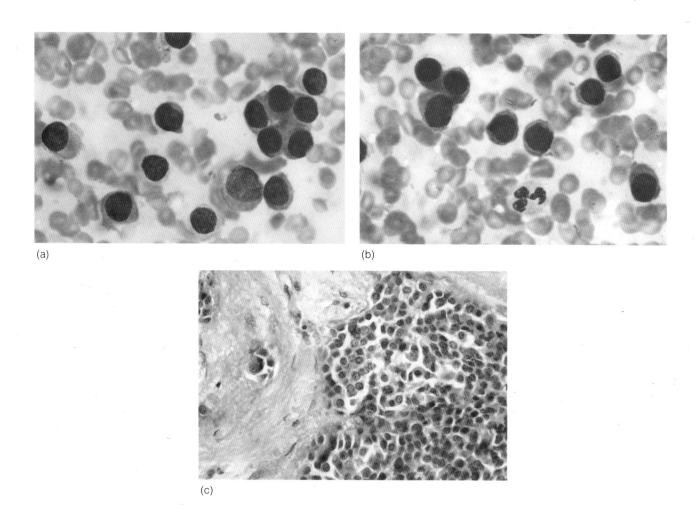

(a)

(b)

(c)

CASE 9

The cells in Case 9 were found in cyst fluid aspirated from a recurrent cyst in the right breast from a lady aged 51. She had had cysts aspirated previously from the same area of the breast on four separate occasions over the previous 18 months.

Figure 4.9a shows that the cells are very large and pleomorphic but present a syncytial appearance. The nuclei themselves show a dispersed chromatin pattern with absent nucleoli. The edges of the cluster present a rather fibrillary appearance. In another field (Fig. 4.9b) the syncytial and multinucleated aspects of this cluster are well shown. To the left three elongated cells are present with rather loose cytoplasm. Although very alarming these cells do not indicate malignancy. It is likely that they are metaplastic as a consequence of the repeated cyst aspiration. Twelve years later this patient is well with no evidence of carcinoma.

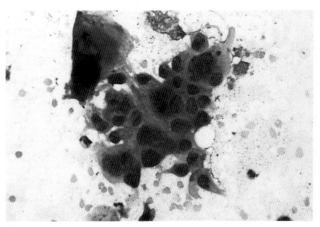

(a)

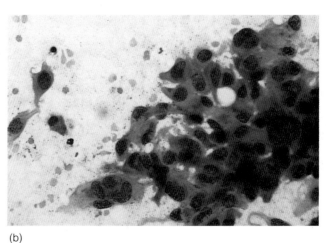

(b)

CASE 10

A lady aged 42 had had DCIS with a small focus of invasive carcinoma diagnosed on excision biopsy ten months previously. One month later she had a re-excision and axillary dissection as the previous sample was thought to be incompletely removed. A further area of carcinoma *in situ* was identified. The axillary nodes showed no evidence of metastatic carcinoma. She was therefore subsequently given radiotherapy and six months later an area of thickening was aspirated.

Figure 4.10a is a low-power photomicrograph of a loose aggregate of large apocrine-like cells having pleomorphic nuclei. A few intranuclear vacuoles are present in the centre of the field. These cells are certainly abnormal and raise the suspicion of malignancy. Similar cells are seen in the left of Fig. 4.10b. These appear to be adherent to a leash of benign-looking duct epithelial cells that appear attached to a central capillary. Figure 4.10c is a very large, slightly distorted cell with possibly two nuclei, one of which contains a large nucleolus. Surrounding this there are reactive nuclei present. In Fig. 4.10d a cell with lacy cytoplasm is present. The cell has two nuclei both of which have prominent nucleoli. Although aprocrine-like, they are very atypical. In the upper part of the field an irregular nucleus is seen with a central vacuole. The cytological appearances were suspicious of recurrent DCIS and excision by biopsy was performed.

At low power (Fig. 4.10e), microcystic structures are present outlined by similar cells to those seen in the cytology specimen. In the lower part of the photomicrograph some normal small breast ducts are present.

At higher power (Fig. 4.10f), the apocrine-like nature of these cells is apparent as well as multi-nucleation and prominent nucleoli. These are radiotherapy effects and there is no evidence of recurrent carcinoma.

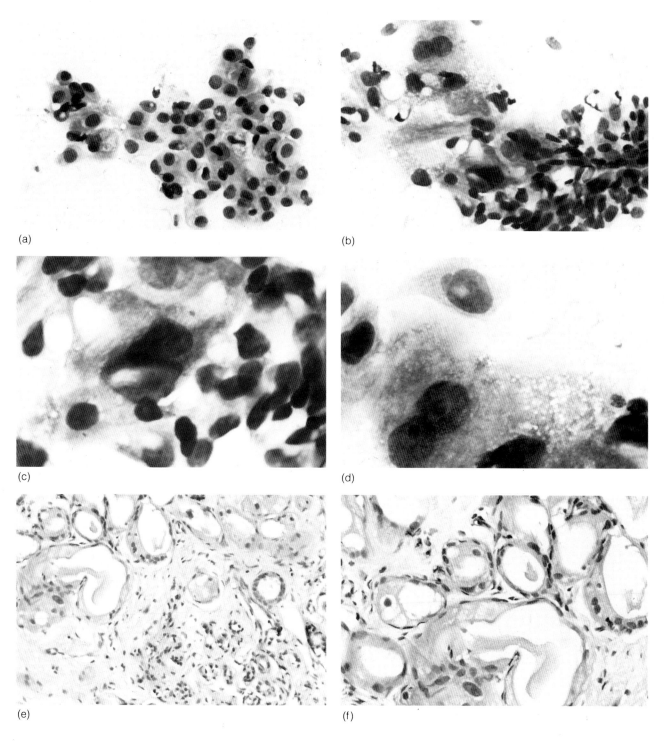

(a)

(b)

(c)

(d)

(e)

(f)

CASE 11

The cells in Fig. 4.11a were aspirated from a breast cyst in a 48-year-old woman. She had a palpable lump and 9.5 ml of rather turbid fluid was removed. The cells in the deposit are very large and have eccentric nuclei. The cytoplasm has a lattice-like appearance and there is pink-staining fibrillary material in the background.

In Fig. 4.11b two large cells are present: one is multinucleated and the other has a lobed nucleus. They show an apocrine appearance although the multinucleated cell may be a facultative histiocyte. The important feature is the similarity of the chro-

matin structure which is generally bland.

The cells in benign cysts often present alarming appearances. Often they appear very atypical as in this case which was reported as 'atypical, C3'. In the event the aspirate procedure 'cured' the patient and no palpable abnormality remained. She is well 14 years later. It is important that the cytopathologist knows that the specimen is cyst fluid. When slides are presented to the laboratory the clinician may omit this information which can lead to a false diagnosis of malignancy and the consequent anxiety.

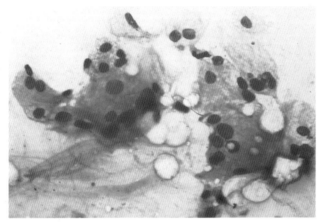

(a)

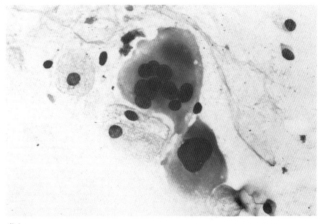

(b)

CASE 12

The cells from Case 12 were aspirated from a solid mobile lump in the left breast of a lady aged 37. The smears were only moderately cellular but included groups and single cells that were atypical. In Fig. 4.12a, taken at high power, a group of cells with five nuclei is seen on the right of the photomicrograph. There is obvious nuclear border irregularity and a suggestion of moulding as well as intranuclear vacuolation. On the left of the picture there is a small round bare nucleus and another one adjacent having a notch in the nuclear border. In retrospect these are probably myoepithelial cells but at the time of diagnosis the cell cluster was thought to be 'very suspicious of carcinoma, C4'.

In Fig. 4.12b a sheet is present showing cells with rounded large nuclei (compare with the red blood cells in the background). The striking feature here is monomorphism and it is not evident that there are two cell types in this cluster. The patient proceeded to excision biopsy as a consequence of the cytological report. The histology revealed a fibroadenoma. Figure 4.12c shows the pericanicular pattern of a fibroadenoma at high-power magnification. The epithelial clusters appear similar to those seen in the aspirate. The cytology was reviewed and the surgeon reassured that the cytological appearances were compatible with the histology and that no carcinoma had been overlooked.

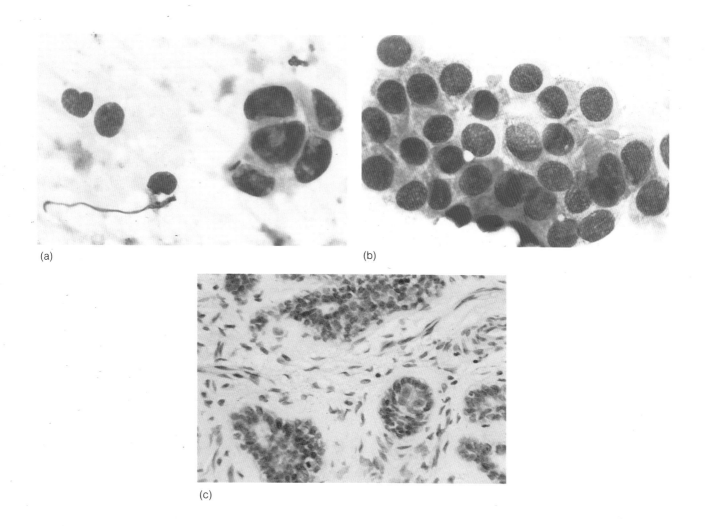

(a)

(b)

(c)

CASE 13

The cells aspirated from a carcinoma from a lady aged 57 show the familiar criteria of malignancy. In Fig. 4.13a one cell in the centre of the photomicrograph contains numerous basophilic granules in the cytoplasm. In Fig. 4.13b granules are seen in several other cells from the same patient. They appear to vary slightly in size and are numerous. Figure 4.13c is the histology section stained with chromogranin. Several cells are positive.

The identification of neuroendocrine granules in cytological specimens has no significance so far as therapy is concerned but, occasionally, it can be very helpful in differentiating a proliferative benign lesion from carcinoma. When atypical cells are present that do not totally conform to the malignant criteria, the finding of basophilic granules in a few cells can clinch a malignant diagnosis.

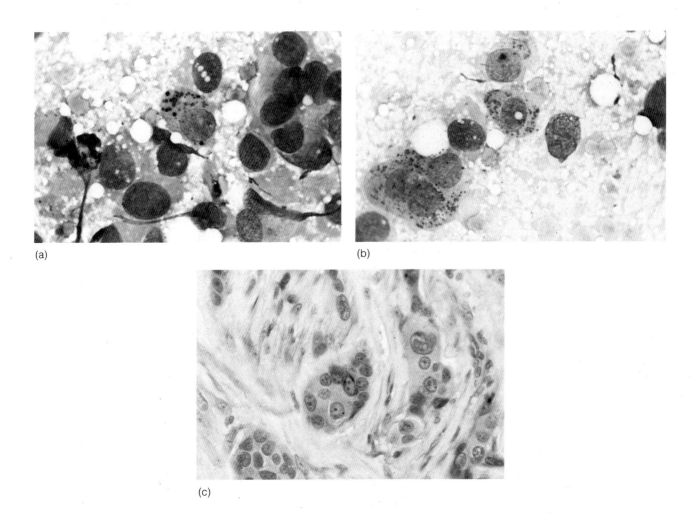

(a)

(b)

(c)

CASE 14

Figure 4.14a shows the cells present in a bloody nipple aspirate from a woman aged 62. Although rather obscured, the clustering of the cells can be identified and a few have elongated large atypical nuclei. Similar cells are illustrated in Fig. 4.14b and some very large nuclei (which can be compared with the size of the red blood cells) are present, especially in the lower central part of the photomicrograph. These appearances were reported as 'suspicious of malignancy, C4' and a periareolar mass was excised. The histology (Fig. 4.14c), showed a papillary lesion having a disorderly architecture. This was diagnosed as papillary duct carcinoma *in situ*, of low grade malignancy.

The difficulty in interpreting cells found in nipple aspirates is to differentiate between papilloma and papillary carcinoma. This is not straightforward and there is a histopathological range between these two lesions which tends to overlap. Unless the cells are categorically malignant it is wisest to be circumspect with the diagnosis and issue an equivocal report.

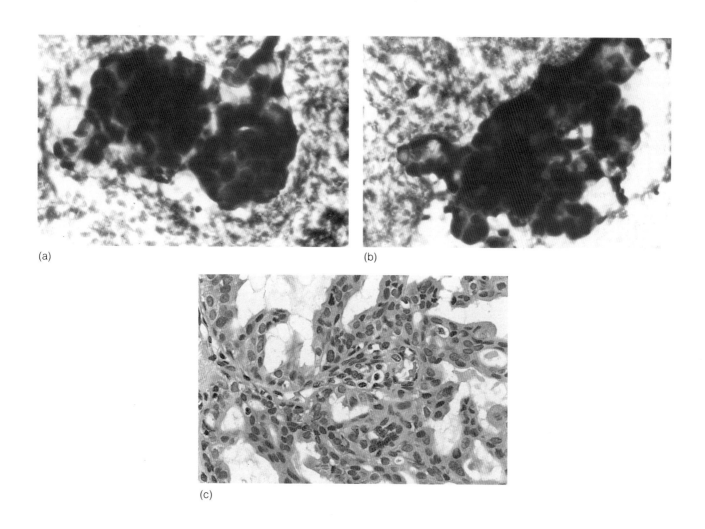

(a)

(b)

(c)

CASE 15

Figure 4.15a is a high-power photomicrograph showing neuroendocrine granules in a carcinoma. The cells are large and pleomorphic with prominent nucleoli and centrally the characteristic basophil granules are seen. Figure 4.15b is another field from the same case showing more cytoplasmic granules. The variation in size is well shown.

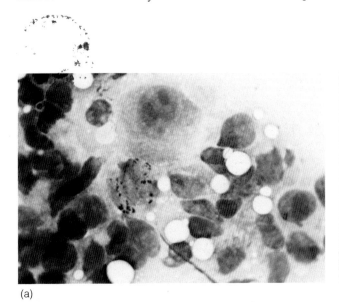

(a)

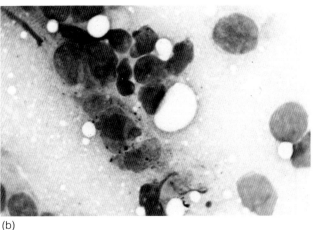

(b)

CASE 16

A patient, aged 52 years, had a lump in the upper outer quadrant of the right breast which had been present for about 18 months. Clinically, it was smooth and mobile. Mammographic examination was unhelpful. The needle aspirate specimen was cellular and was reported as showing 'clusters, pairs and single benign duct epithelial cells. No evidence of malignancy, C2'. Although this was thought to be a benign mass probably a fibroadenoma, it was thought wisest to remove it on account of the patient's age. This advice was resisted and the mass was not removed.

At subsequent visits there was no change in the nature of the lump and the patient still would not agree to an operation. However, 19 months after the first visit it was thought the lump had increased in size and it was excised.

Figure 4.16a is an aspirate from the original specimen which shows a tight cluster of monomorphic cells, a pair of myoepithelial cells and other single cells with 'bare nuclei'. These appearances were thought to show the cytological features of a benign aspirate. A cluster (Fig. 4.16b) is seen at high-power photomicrography in which two populations of cells are present. The larger cells show individual monomorphism and have elongated-shaped nuclei and intracytoplasmic vacuoles. They are also very large. In the top left-hand corner smaller oval-shaped pyknotic nuclei are present which were thought to be myoepithelial cells. Similar cells are present in Fig. 4.16c including those that are large and irregular, and a 'bare nucleus' that is seen on the left-hand side of the picture. Figure 4.16d is another field showing cells with large irregular nuclei. Pleomorphism and nuclear border irregularity is seen. Figure 4.16e is a low-power photomicrograph of the histological specimen which showed a low grade, grade 1 infiltrating ductal carcinoma. At higher power (Fig. 4.16f), the features of the infiltrating carcinoma cells can be compared with the cytological specimen. This case is one of a missed carcinoma. The carcinoma is low grade and well differentiated, but in retrospect features sugges-

tive of carcinoma in the needle aspirate specimen should have been recognized. It would not have been possible in this case to have given a certain diagnosis of malignancy owing to the presence of undoubted myoepithelial cell nuclei both within clusters and in pairs. In practical terms, had an equivocal cytological diagnosis been given, excision biopsy would have been undertaken sooner.

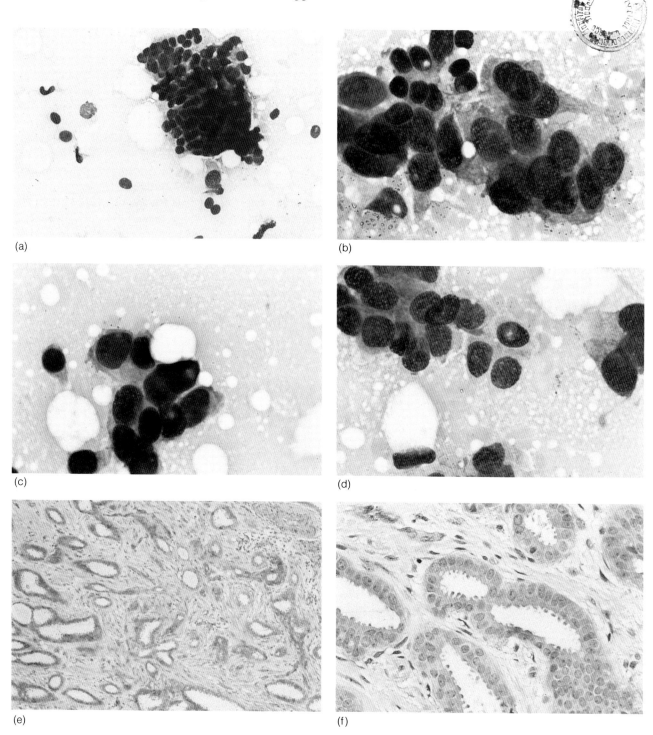

(a)

(b)

(c)

(d)

(e)

(f)

CASE 17

A lady presented with a five-week history of a 4 cm clinical carcinoma in the upper central part of the left breast. She was aged 46 years and was premenopausal. It was decided to treat her with primary chemotherapy (neo-adjuvant therapy) consisting of six courses of CMF (cyclophosphamide, methotrexate and 5-fluorouracil) to be followed by elective surgery. Fine needle aspiration and Tru-cut biopsy were undertaken.

Figure 4.17a is a very low-power view of the needle aspirate. Large clusters are present with frayed edges and scattered cells in between. In Fig. 4.17b the dyshesion of the cluster can be seen as well as the presence of one population of cells. At high power (Fig. 4.17c), a monomorphic group of cells is seen with absent cytoplasm and round or oval nuclei. Although there is some nuclear moulding, there is little nuclear border irregularity. The Giemsa stain provides the cells with a pale-blue hue.

The size of the cells can be gauged from the diameter of a rather degenerate polymorph present in Fig. 4.17d. Although in the cluster a few nuclei resemble myoepithelial cells, it is generally unreliable to identify these in cell clusters. These cytological appearances are characteristic of carcinoma, despite the comparative lack of pleomorphism and the rather bland appearance of the chromatin. Note that nucleoli are also largely absent. The Tru-cut biopsy (Fig. 4.17e) shows a low grade infiltrating carcinoma. This tumour proved very sensitive to chemotherapy and after one dose the mass had shrunk to half its original size. After three doses no definite lump could be palpated. This patient proceeded to formal excision of the tumour area when a fibrotic mass was identified in which only a few microscopic foci of residual carcinoma were present.

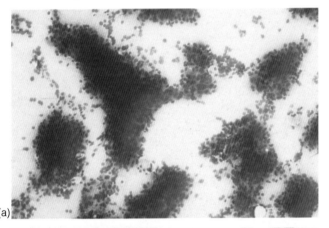
(a)

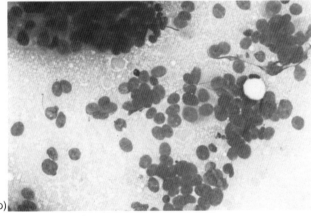
(b)

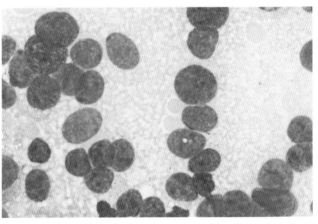
(c)

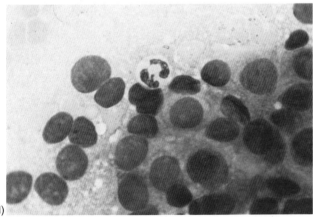
(d)

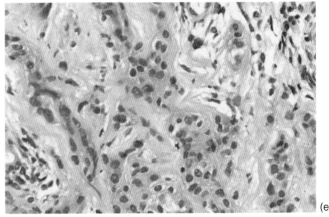
(e)

CASE 18

A post-menopausal 59-year-old lady had a wide local excision of a carcinoma in the left breast followed by radiotherapy. Five years later an area of thickening was found in the region of the former carcinoma and a needle aspirate undertaken.

A moderately cellular sample was aspirated and the photomicrograph (Fig. 4.18a) taken at high power, shows very atypical cells with some pleomorphism and nuclear border irregularity. In other fields rather more worrying appearances were seen consisting of large very pleomorphic nuclei and prominent nucleoli in a dispersed cluster (Fig.

4.18b). Figure 4.18c shows similar highly atypical cells. These appearances were thought to be 'highly suspicious of recurrent carcinoma, C4'. Excision of the thickened area was undertaken. The histology (Fig. 4.18d) shows radiotherapy effects and no carcinoma. There is a group of distorted epithelial cells resembling apocrine metaplasia, but showing many nuclei with very large nucleoli. This case illustrates the difficulties of interpreting needle aspirate specimens following radiotherapy even five years previously. Ten years after the diagnosis of her carcinoma she is well with no sign of recurrence.

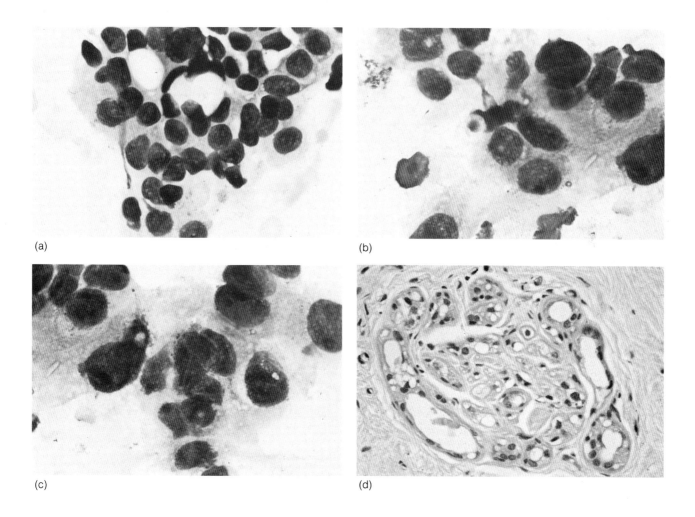

(a)

(b)

(c)

(d)

CASE 19

This patient is aged 27 and the needle aspirate was misinterpreted as benign. Despite this, the mass was excised and it showed an infiltrating grade 2 ductal carcinoma.

At low power (Fig. 4.19a), the cells are mainly in tight clusters similar to the pattern seen in a fibroadenoma. At medium power (Fig. 4.19b), rather rounded nuclei were identified resembling myoepithelial cell nuclei. At high power under oil-immersion (Fig. 4.19c), the true nature of these cells is revealed. Although small they are extremely atypical and show a variation in size, nuclear moulding and are all one type of cell. They certainly indicate carcinoma. Elsewhere, mitoses were pre-

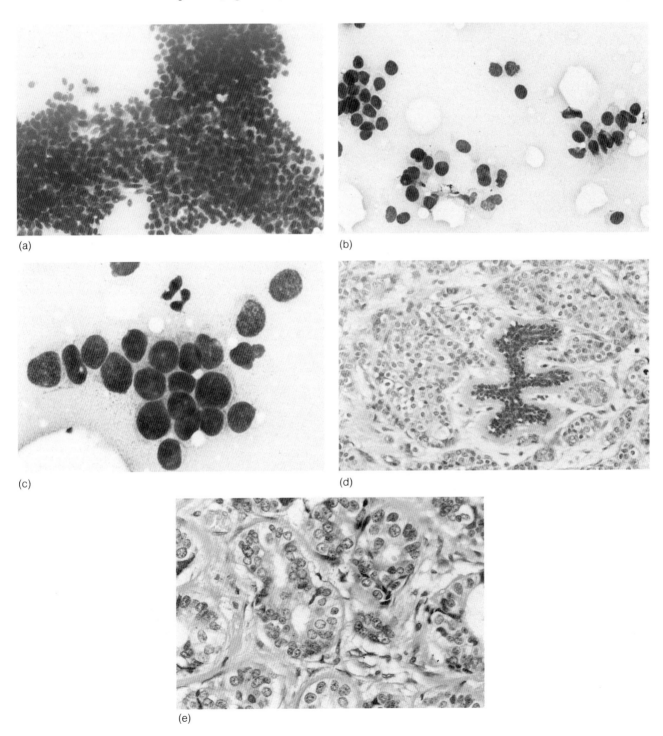

(a)

(b)

(c)

(d)

(e)

sent. This specimen was misinterpreted as a fibroadenoma.

The histology (Fig. 4.19d) shows an infiltrating carcinoma surrounding a normal breast duct. At high power (Fig. 4.19e), the histological appearances of the nuclei can be compared with those seen in the cytology, Fig. 4.19c. Aspiration cytodiagnosis of breast lumps in young women should never be omitted. Clinically a carcinoma will resemble a fibroadenoma and mammography is usually not done. So often, needle aspiration provides the first clue to the true nature of the tumour.

CASE 20

A patient received adjuvant chemotherapy and radiotherapy following excision of a poorly differentiated carcinoma. Seven months later she felt some vague thickening in the area of the previous excision and a fine needle aspirate was taken.

At low power several elongated groups of very large cells, stained by the Papanicolaou technique, were seen (Fig. 4.20a). At high power (Fig. 4.20b), their size can be compared to the adjacent red blood cells and the clumped chromatin pattern and prominent nucleoli seen. In Fig. 4.20c a bizarre-shaped nucleus is present with very clumped nuclear chromatin. These appearances are those of radiotherapy effects and should not be regarded as malignant.

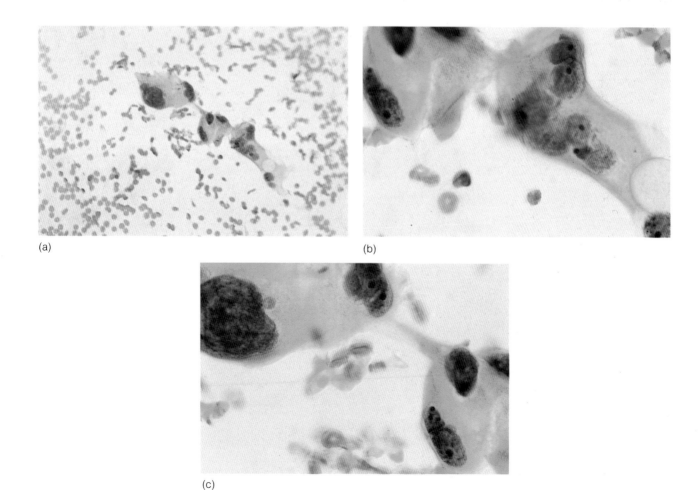

(a)

(b)

(c)

CASE 21

A patient, aged 45, presented with an area of indistinct nodularity in the lower inner quadrant of the right breast. Aspiration cytodiagnosis was reported 'highly suspicious of malignancy, C3'. Largely on account of this she proceeded to wide local excision.

At high power (Fig. 4.21a), the cells all appear highly atypical. There is extensive nuclear moulding, intracytoplasmic vacuolation and nuclear border irregularity. Although the nuclei are small and with absent nucleoli, these appearances were thought probably to be carcinoma. Other cells were larger with marked nuclear border irregularity (Fig. 4.21b). Although these perhaps show evidence of degeneration they have highly abnormal nuclei. In Fig. 4.21c again very atypical cells are evident. A neutrophil is present at the lower left-hand corner of the photomicrograph to provide a scale. The cells are overlapping in Fig. 4.21d and their true appearance can only be assessed better by focusing through the cluster.

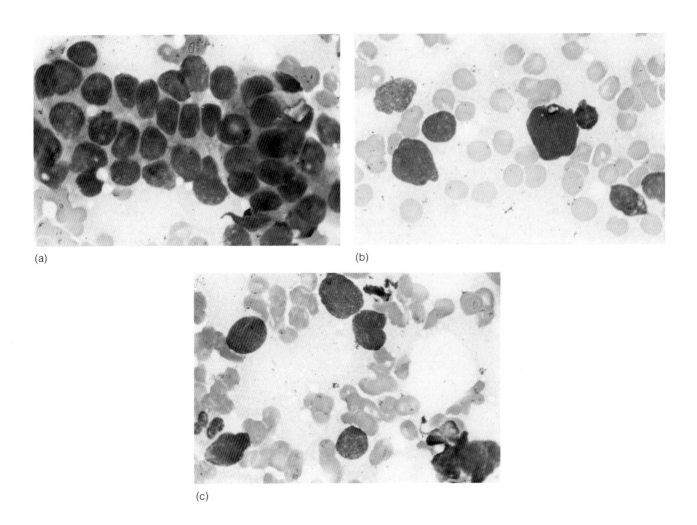

(a)

(b)

(c)

There is marked pleomorphism, nuclear moulding and nuclear border irregularity. The histology (Fig. 4.21e) showed no evidence of carcinoma. However, there was a proliferative lesion present that had a variety of patterns including apocrine metaplasia. At high power in Fig. 4.21f, atypical apocrine cells are seen with prominent nucleoli and abundant cytoplasm. All the tissue was sectioned.

This case illustrates what is so often found when trying to reconcile the cytological and histological appearances. The cells in the cytology smear do not really look apocrine and yet in the section this was the area of concern. The explanation for the discrepancy must lie in the different methods of preparation of the two specimens; certainly the area of atypical apocrine metaplasia in the sections caused much concern. One year later this lady is well with no sign of carcinoma.

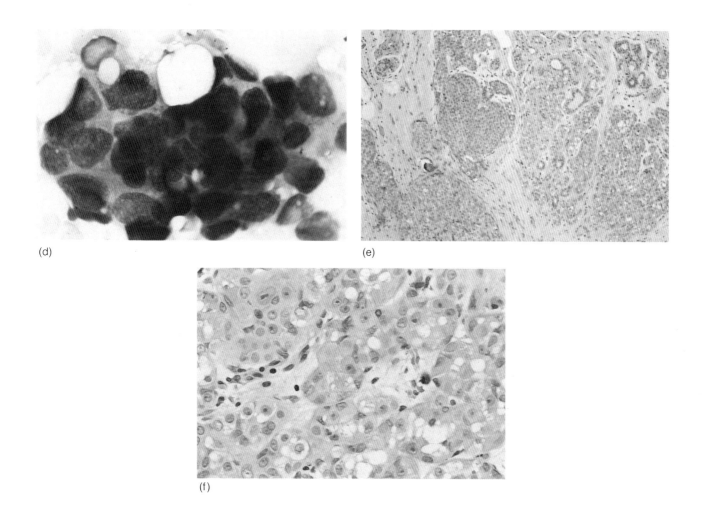

(d)

(e)

(f)

CASE 22

A patient, aged 72, had a clinical carcinoma in the left breast confirmed at mammography. She also had extensive alcoholic cirrhosis and was a poor anaesthetic risk.

At low power the aspirate is seen to be a good-quality well-smeared cellular sample showing a capillary blood vessel at the left-hand side of the photomicrograph. The clusters are dyshesive and at this power a double population of nuclei can be identified (Fig. 4.22a). At high power (Fig. 4.22b), small cells are seen, about the size of lymphocytes showing nuclear moulding and some variation in size. To the right of the photomicrograph a cuboidal epithelial cell is present. Figure 4.22c shows crowding, nuclear moulding and pleomorphism with possibly two epithelial cell nuclei at the lower border of the cluster.

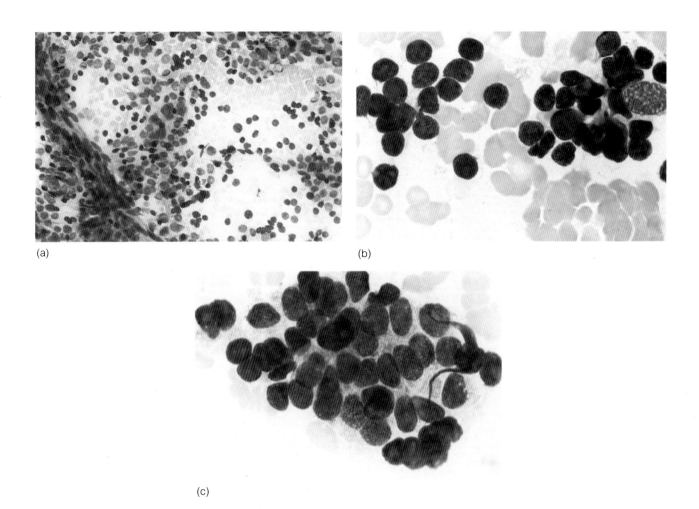

(a)

(b)

(c)

In Fig. 4.22d there is one single very large highly atypical nucleus with a central nucleolus that is about the size of a red blood cell. Another large very atypical cell and a small round one showing a 'nuclear nipple' are shown in Fig. 4.22e.

This specimen was difficult to interpret and the temptation was to issue a report highly suspicious of malignancy. However, taking into account the other two components of the 'triple approach' a diagnosis of carcinoma, C5 was issued. Had these appearances been present in a younger woman with equivocal clinical and radiological findings a more circumspect diagnosis would have been appropriate. Because of the atraumatic nature of this technique, cytopathologists are often asked to confirm other investigative findings using less than perfect material.

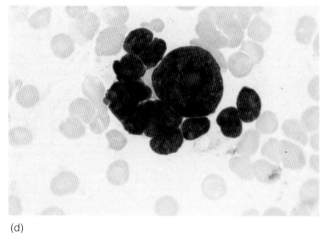

(d)

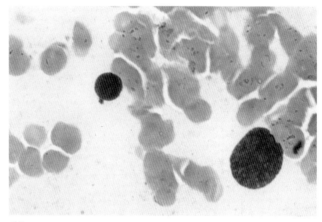

(e)

CASE 23

The specimen is from a 5 cm mass in the upper central area of the right breast in a woman aged 42. Clinically it was firm but not fixed and mammographically it showed a smooth border and was solid on ultrasonography.

The needle aspirate provided a good-quality cellular sample in which a variety of cells were seen (Fig. 4.23a). In this low-power field tight clusters of epithelial cells are present as well as histiocytes, probable myoepithelial cell nuclei and foam cells. At high power two populations of nuclei are apparent, the larger with vesicular oval nuclei indicating cuboidal epithelial cells and the smaller pyknotic nuclei which include one 'pair' which are

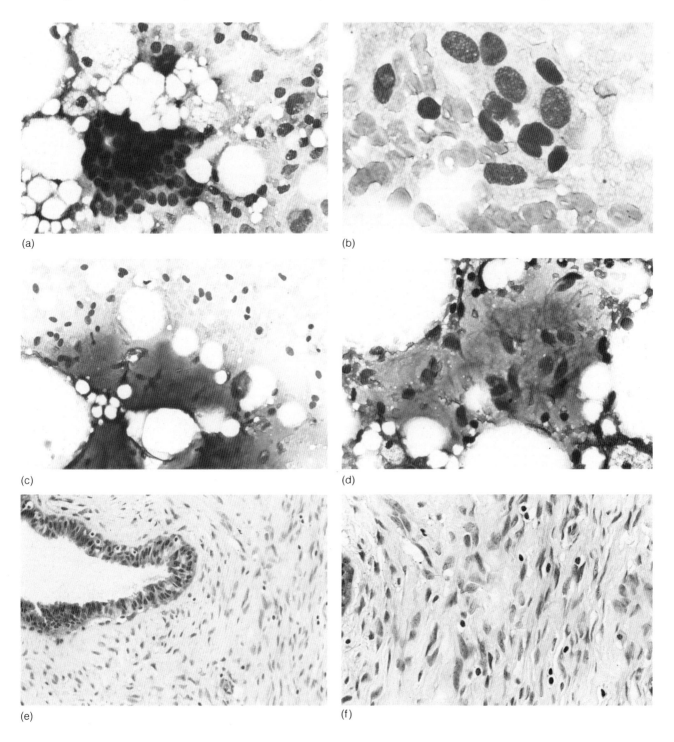

(a)

(b)

(c)

(d)

(e)

(f)

myoepithelial (Fig. 4.23b). Elsewhere metachromatic staining stroma is present which shows a bright purple colour (Fig. 4.23c). Adjacent to this area are single and pairs of myoepithelial nuclei. In Fig. 4.23d larger spindly cells were present within the metachromatic staining stroma. This appearance provides the clue to the diagnosis. The histology (Fig. 4.23e) showed a low grade phyllodes tumour in which the epithelial clefts were surrounded by a cellular spindle cell stroma. At higher power the cellular nature of this stroma is evident (Fig. 4.23f). Note that within the stroma there are scattered myoepithelial nuclei.

CASE 24

A patient, aged 55, had been attending a breast screening unit for 10 years. At one visit to the clinic a discrete 1.5 cm lesion was found in the left breast. This was suspicious on mammography. A needle aspirate was taken. At low power, discrete rounded clusters were identified with generally regular edges (Fig. 4.24a). At higher power, the regularity of the cluster borders is more easily seen and large rather monomorphic nuclei are present showing some degree of fragmentation (Fig. 4.24b).

In Fig. 4.24c more atypical cells were identified showing nuclear moulding, pleomorphism and nuclear border irregularity. On the basis of these appearances a report was issued 'carcinoma present, C5'. The histology (Fig. 4.24d) of the excised lesion reflects the cytological appearances. This is a grade one well-differentiated infiltrating ductal carcinoma in which clustering is a feature of the pattern. There is little cellular pleomorphism. Note that well-differentiated low grade carcinoma can be difficult to diagnose in an aspirate specimen. However, attention to nuclear detail, seen best under oil-immersion microscopy, can successfully make the diagnosis.

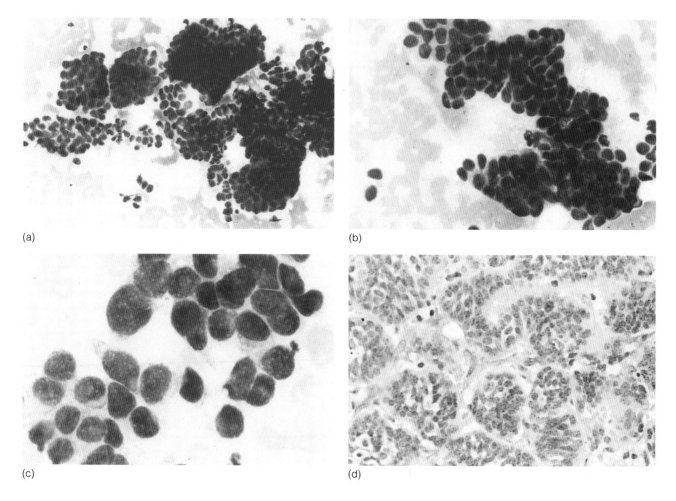

(a)

(b)

(c)

(d)

CASE 25

A patient, aged 28 years, had had three fibroadeno-mas removed over the course of the previous four years. At recent examination another mobile lump was palpated and aspirated.

At low power part of an 'antler-like' sheet of cells is seen, with scattered single cells in the lower right-hand part of the photomicrograph, Fig. 4.25a. In Fig. 4.25b two cuboidal epithelial cell nuclei are identified as well as six myoepithelial nuclei, two of which are opposed pole-to-pole. Figure 4.25c shows the rather atypical cuboidal epithelial cells which show a degree of pleomorphism. A single

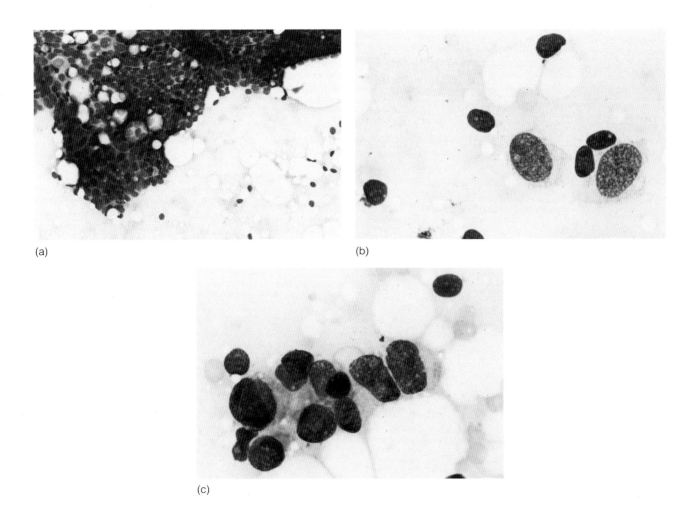

(a)

(b)

(c)

myoepithelial cell within the group is seen. In Fig. 4.25d there are three pairs of myoepithelial cell nuclei which are found in profusion in aspirates from fibroadenomas. The excision biopsy specimen confirmed a fibraoadenoma (Fig. 4.25e). Although in this case the diagnosis was straightforward fibro-

adenomas have been misdiagnosed as carcinomas on aspiration cytology. The epithelial clefts often show reactive features but the clue to the diagnosis lies in the large number of myoepithelial cell nuclei present.

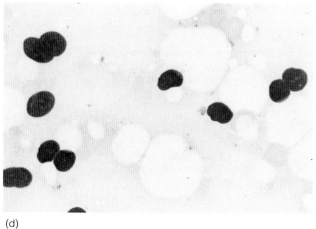
(d)

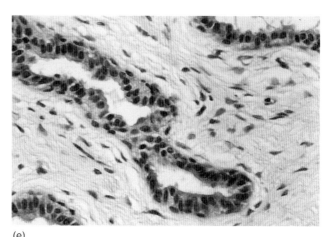
(e)

REFERENCES

1. Cytology subgroup of the National Coordinating Committee for Breast Cancer Screening Pathology, (eds. C. A. Wells, I. O. Ellis, H. D. Zakhour and A. R. Wilson) (1994) Guidelines for cytology procedures and reporting on fine needle aspirates of the breast. *Cytology* **5**, 316–34.

2. Trott, P. A. and Walsh, P. (1993) Paintings in Cytology. *Cytopathology*, **4**, supplement 1, 12.

3. Papanicolaou, G. N. (1954) *Atlas of Exfoliative Cytology*, Harvard University Press for the Commonwealth Fund, Cambridge, Mass.

4. Spriggs, A. I. (1957) *The Cytology of Effusions*, Heinemann, London.

5. Uncommon lesions

Clive A. Wells

INTRODUCTION

Every so often fine needle aspiration will be performed on uncommon lesions occurring in the breast. As experience in breast cytology has increased more unusual lesions have been aspirated that have been correlated with their counterpart histopathology. Furthermore, the introduction of the UK National Health Service Breast Screening Programme has resulted in the biopsy of small impalpable mammographic abnormalities, the interpretation of which has provided new challenges for histopathologists. Stereotactic needle aspiration has provided cytopathological specimens from these lesions and experience is accumulating concerning their cytological interpretation.

The lesions to be discussed in this section are shown in Table 5.1 where they are subdivided into those which are primarily epithelial, those which are myoepithelial or stromal and those which are soft tissue lesions that occur elsewhere in the body.

EPITHELIAL LESIONS

Juvenile papillomatosis

Juvenile papillomatosis (sometimes known as Swiss cheese disease) [1] is characterized by multiple apocrine cysts, foamy macrophages, regular epithelial hyperplasia and sclerosing adenosis. It is a localized breast tumour of young women, first described as a clinicopathological entity in 1980. There is a link with breast cancer, in that many cases have a positive family history, but there is no good evidence that the lesion itself is precancerous [2].

The cytological features are not very different from fibrocystic change with hyperplasia but, due to the extensive nature of the hyperplasia, the smears may be very cellular and sometimes three-dimensional clusters of epithelial cells may be present. In addition, streaming of spindle cells from sclerosing adenosis, apocrine metaplastic cells, foam cells and benign bipolar bare nuclei may be seen. It is not usually possible to make a definitive diagnosis of this condition unless some prior history is known but it is necessary to be aware of the combination of features to avoid over-diagnosis of the hyperplastic clusters (Fig. 5.1).

Tubular adenoma

Mammary tubular adenoma, like fibroadenoma of which it is a variant, occurs in young women. It is a well-circumscribed lesion, yellow on cut section with a soft consistency composed of adenomatous tubules surrounded by myoepithelial cells. The cytological features resemble fibroadenoma with fewer bare nuclei and it is possible to see occasional benign tubules in some cases (Fig. 5.2).

Table 5.1 Uncommon lesions

Epithelial lesions	Myoepithelial/stromal lesions	Soft tissue lesions
Juvenile papillomatosis	Phyllodes tumour	Fibromatosis and nodular fasciitis
Adenomas	Nodular sclerosing adenosis	Schwannoma
Gynaecomastia	Adenomyoepithelioma	Granular cell tumour
Apocrine adenosis	Pleomorphic adenoma	Lymphoma/chloroma
Microglandular adenosis		Hamartoma
Collagenous spherulosis		Haemangiosarcoma
Atypical hyperplasia		Stromal sarcoma
Tubular carcinoma		Haemangiopericytoma
Apocrine carcinoma		
Squamous carcinoma		
Adenoid cystic carcinoma		
Neuroendocrine carcinoma		

Ductal adenoma

Ductal adenoma was first described in 1984 by Azzopardi and Salm [3]. It is an intraductal lesion found in medium-sized ducts and is composed of sclerosed adenomatous tubules with myoepithelial cells set within dense fibrous tissue. Apocrine metaplasia may be present. Some pathologists regard the lesion as one of the variants of the complex sclerosing lesion.

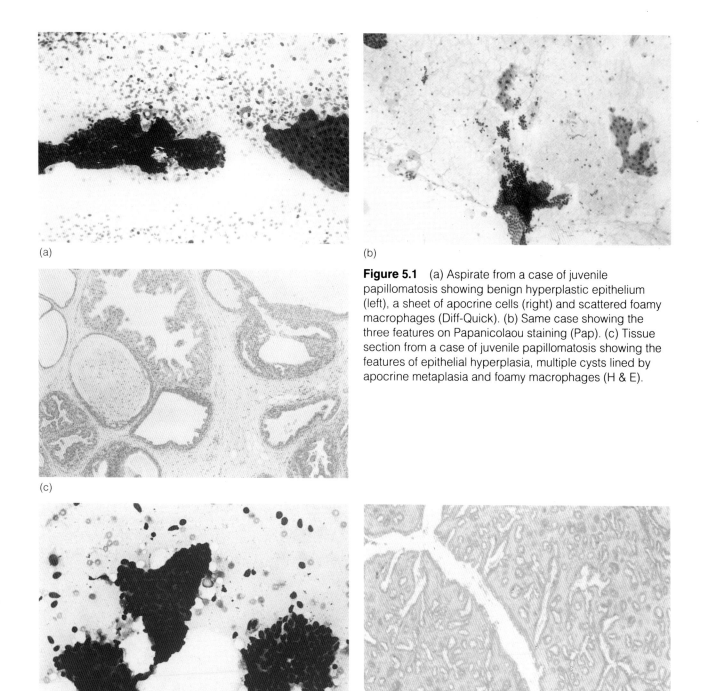

(a)

(b)

Figure 5.1 (a) Aspirate from a case of juvenile papillomatosis showing benign hyperplastic epithelium (left), a sheet of apocrine cells (right) and scattered foamy macrophages (Diff-Quick). (b) Same case showing the three features on Papanicolaou staining (Pap). (c) Tissue section from a case of juvenile papillomatosis showing the features of epithelial hyperplasia, multiple cysts lined by apocrine metaplasia and foamy macrophages (H & E).

(c)

(a)

(b)

Figure 5.2 (a) Aspirate from a case of tubular adenoma showing compact clusters of benign epithelial cells and bare nuclei indistinguishable from fibroadenoma (Diff-Quick). (b) Tissue section from the same case showing small tubules set within fibrous stroma (H & E).

The cytopathology of this condition has not been described in detail in the literature but one of the two cases the author has seen presented diagnostic difficulty and led to a report of atypia (Fig. 5.3). The cytology specimen showed compact clusters of cells with overlapping, but often with two cell types (epithelial cells and smaller spindle cells with some myoepithelial features). Tubules may be present and these should not be mistaken for tubular carcinoma. The cells may be nucleolated but are usually round or oval in shape. Fibrous tissue is often present. 'Naked' nuclei, though present may be scanty. Apocrine metaplastic cells were seen.

Nipple adenoma

This neoplasm which is common in the fifth decade [10], may be present clinically as a reddened eczematous-appearing nipple, simulating Paget's disease of the nipple. Other patients notice bloody or serious nipple discharge, pain or a lump beneath the nipple. Histology of this entity shows florid proliferation of papillary fronds and solid cellular areas. The papillary areas are composed of delicate branching vascular connective tissue stalks covered by cuboidal epithelial cells resting on a myoepithelial layer (Figs 6.20 and 6.21). The varying clinical presentations and histological features of several cases, including ones showing squamous epithelium lining tubules, are well documented [11, 12]. Some cases are associated with breast carcinoma [13] either with malignant changes developing in the benign lesion or a coincidental cancer in the same breast.

Nipple smears in this condition vary in cellularity. They contain erythrocytes, debris, foamy macrophages and clusters of benign ductal cells. These may show mild pleomorphism but no definite features of malignancy.

Gynaecomastia

Gynaecomastia (Fig. 5.4), a condition of the male

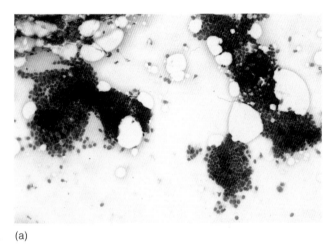

(a)

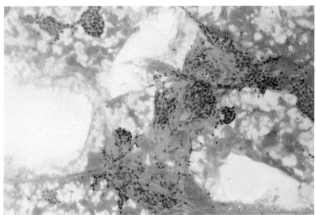

(b)

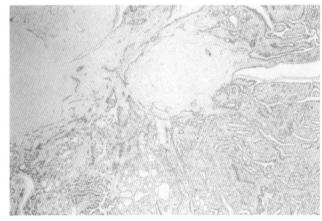

(c)

Figure 5.3 (a) Aspirate from a case of ductal adenoma of the breast showing hyperplastic clusters of benign epithelial cells but with some more pleomorphic dissociated epithelial cells. Note also the bare nuclei in the background (Diff-Quick). (b) The same case on Papanicolaou staining showing benign epithelium and stromal tissue. (c) Tissue section from the same case showing proliferated tubular glands and sclerosis with entrapped glands in the central scar. Note also the apocrine metaplasia (H & E).

breast, is characterized in its early stages by epithelial proliferation and budding with sometimes a low papillary pattern within the ducts. The ducts are surrounded by loose connective tissue reminiscent of lobular connective tissue in the female breast. Aspirates of cases of gynaecomastia can be markedly cellular with large sheets of epithelial cells, sometimes containing cells with nuclear atypia and occasionally mitotic figures. There are reports in the literature of the diagnosis of carcinoma in cases of gynaecomastia [6, 7], usually when the condition is in the early or active phase. The atypical cells with mitotic figures are presumably from the hyperplastic epithelium in the ducts. There may also be some dissociation but this is mild and the cells do not usually show an abnormal chromatin pattern although they may show some anisonucleosis with hyperchromasia. The most striking features leading to the diagnosis are the presence of tightly cohesive groups and three-dimensional clusters of epithelial cells that have a small amount of cytoplasm. Chemotherapeutic drugs may accentuate the hyperplastic changes [8].

Apocrine adenosis

Apocrine adenosis [9] mimics carcinoma in cytological smears and can be difficult to interpret on histology. Also because of the marked cytological atypia of the pleomorphic apocrine cells (Fig 5.5), atypical apocrine cells in fine needle aspirates should always be interpreted with caution [10]. In the presence of bare nuclei even bizarre aprocrine cells may not be malignant and clues can be gained from the appearance of the cells in the epithelial clumps. These show two cell types, atypical apocrine cells and spindle-shaped cells. These appearances are especially marked in cases occurring in sclerosing adenosis.

Microglandular adenosis

Microglandular adenosis is characterized histologically by single-layered tubules set in fat and surrounded by basement membrane but with no discernible myoepithelial layer. Cytologically it may

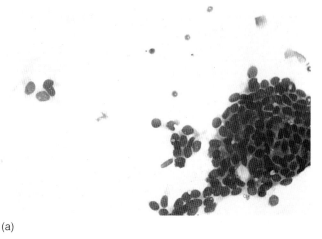

(a)

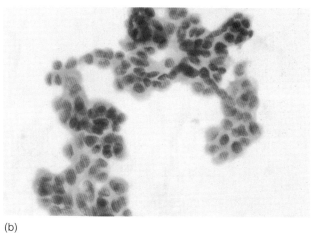

(b)

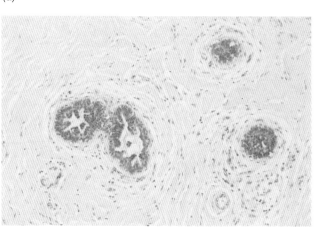

(c)

Figure 5.4 (a) Aspirate from a case of gynaecomastia showing a hyperplastic epithelial cluster and bare nuclei (Diff-Quick). (b) Papanicolaou-stained smear from another case showing a more complex papillary cluster but still with two cell types in the cluster (Pap). (c) Tissue section from the same case as (a) showing loose connective tissue surrounding ducts showing a micropapillary type of hyperplasia (H & E).

produce small tubules which can be confused with the tubules seen in cases of tubular carcinoma [11]. Unfortunately it is often seen in association with other lesions such as radial scar and the temptation to diagnose tubular carcinoma may be great. An unequivocal diagnosis of tubular carcinoma should not be made unless there is cytological atypia within the tubular profiles.

Collagenous spherulosis

Collagenous spherulosis can mimic adenoid cystic carcinoma in cytological specimens. It is an extreme form of myoepithelial differentiation in epithelial hyperplasia of the breast and as far as is known, has no premalignant significance. It may be found as an incidental feature in breast aspirates or may be one

of the patterns of hyperplasia found in association with radial scars [12].

The cytological features are those of regular hyperplasia with two cell types surrounding amorphous collagenous material seen as translucent acellular spheres. In contrast to adenoid cystic carcinoma 'bare' nuclei are noted in the background [13] (Fig. 5.6).

Atypical hyperplasia

Atypical hyperplasia may be seen on its own or in association with other lesions especially papilloma, fibrocystic changes and radial scar. It can be divided into two types: atypical lobular hyperplasia (ALH) and atypical ductal hyperplasia (ADH) [14]. As these have different appearances in smears they will be discussed separately.

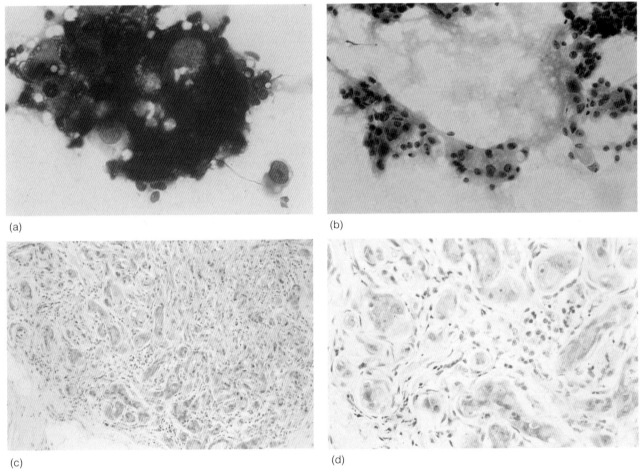

(a)

(b)

(c)

(d)

Figure 5.5 (a) Aspirate from a case of apocrine adenosis showing large highly atypical apocrine cells with pleomorphism of the nuclei (Diff-Quick). (b) Papanicolaou-stained smear from the same case showing atypical apocrine cells (Pap). (c) Tissue section from the same case showing apocrine metaplasia in an area of sclerosing adenosis (H & E). (d) The same area at higher power showing pleomorphism of the apocrine cells (H & E).

Atypical lobular hyperplasia

ALH is a lobular and terminal duct lesion which has been well described by Salhany and Page who have also described the cytological features [15]. The lesion is a partial filling of lobular units by cells resembling those seen in lobular carcinoma *in situ* (LCIS). The process may extend into terminal ducts and carries an increased risk of subsequent malignancy.

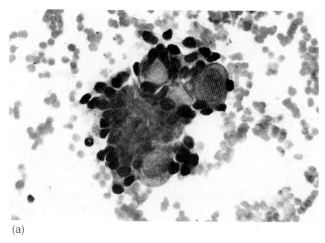

(a)

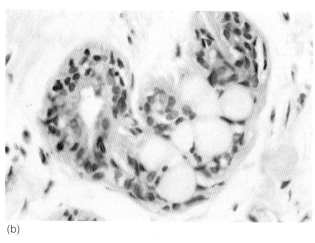

(b)

Figure 5.6 (a) Aspirate from an area of collagenous spherulosis showing purple staining of the basement membrane material of the spherules and surrounding hyperplastic epithelial cells (Diff-Quick). (b) Tissue section from the same case showing hyaline basement membrane material surrounded by flattened myoepithelial cells (H & E).

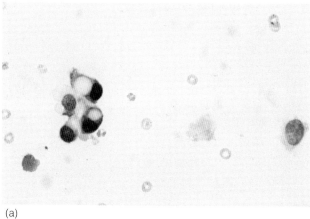

(a)

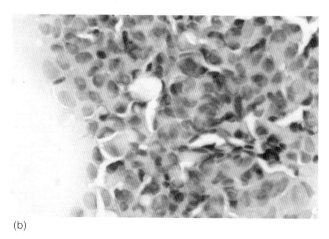

(b)

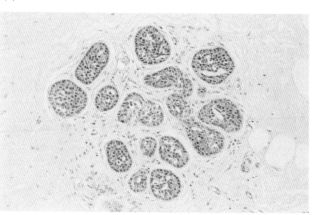

(c)

Figure 5.7 (a) Aspirate from an area of atypical lobular hyperplasia showing small dissociated cells with intracytoplasmic vacuoles and rounded nuclei. These should not be interpreted as unequivocally malignant (Diff-Quick). (b) Papanicolaou stain from the same case showing similar cells to (a) in a mixed group of cells. The atypical cells have small nucleoli. There is a little air drying artefact. (c) Tissue section from the same case showing a lobule affected by the same cells as on the cytology. There is partial filling of the acini and some expansion but the proliferation remains mixed (H & E).

Cytologically (Fig. 5.7), the features are those of dissociation of cells with small rather rounded or squared-off nuclei, often singly or in small groups with nuclear moulding. Sometimes the cells may resemble lobular carcinoma cells with intracytoplasmic lumina seen best on mucin staining where they appear like a 'bullseye' with an alcian blue-stained microvillous membrane and a periodic acid Schiff-stained mucin droplet in the centre. Some pathologists feel the presence of these cells indicates lobular carcinoma, at least *in situ*, but most British pathologists regard ALH as a neoplastic premalignant lesion composed of similar cells to LCIS or invasive lobular carcinoma. The vacuoles are formed due to dilatation of the Golgi apparatus and can be seen well on electron microscopy. ALH can be seen in association with other lesions and so can present confusing appearances on fine needle aspiration smears. It may not be possible to distinguish between ALH, LCIS and even invasive lobular carcinoma in aspirate smears alone.

Atypical ductal hyperplasia

ADH (Fig. 5.8), has become a problem of cytological interpretation with the introduction of stereotactic aspiration. As it can be difficult to distinguish ADH from ductal carcinoma *in situ* (DCIS) on histological grounds it is not surprising that it may also be difficult cytologically.

Most cases of DCIS are of the 'comedo' or large cell type and these do not present a problem as, if they are aspirated, the characteristic features of 'malignant cells' are present along with evidence of necrosis and cell dissociation. The difficulty comes in the aspiration of small cell DCIS of cribriform or micropapillary type. These lesions do not produce necrosis or large numbers of dissociated cells and are mainly recognized by their architectural pattern within the cell clusters. ADH is a similar problem but unlike the monotony of the three-dimensional cell clusters in cribriform DCIS, ADH still shows a biphasic pattern at least in most clusters. They are

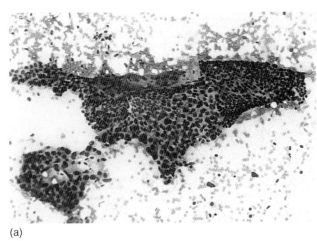

(a)

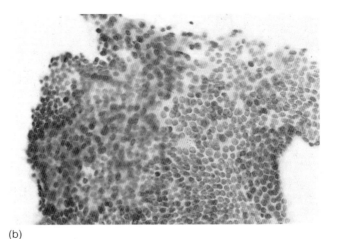

(b)

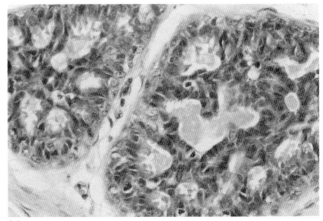

(c)

Figure 5.8 (a) Aspirate from an area of atypical change within a papilloma. There is benign epithelium to the right which merges with epithelium on the left, the cells of which show overtly malignant features. Note also the small bare nuclei in the background. This merging is seen in atypical ductal hyperplasia (Diff-Quick). (b) Similar appearances to Fig. 5.7a in the Papanicolaou stain with the atypical cells showing eosinophilia (Pap). (c) Histology of lesion illustrated in (a) and (b) showing atypical ductal hyperplasia. The duct is expanded and filled by micropapillary structures with luminal spaces of various sizes. The pattern falls short of DCIS.

however, unlike the clusters found in benign disease in that they have a three-dimensional appearance and usually show some cytological atypia, which in some cases is marked.

The literature is not very helpful in the distinction of ADH from benign hyperplasia or small cell DCIS as most reports [16] do not distinguish between those cases of DCIS which are of large cell type and present no diagnostic problem and small cell DCIS. This leads some authors into the mistaken conclusion that the distinction is not a significant problem. With the expansion of stereotaxis there is increasing likelihood that more of these atypical lesions will be sampled.

It is also necessary to remember that this lesion can co-exist with fibrocystic changes, papillomas or radial scar and the radiological appearances may not be characteristic.

Tubular carcinoma

The features of tubular carcinoma on fine needle aspiration are described in detail in the article by Bondeson and Lindholm [17]. These tumours are seen rarely in aspirates from palpable lesions but make up approximately 20 per cent of all tumours in breast screening.

They present as spiculate masses on mammography and may appear similar to radial scars. The cytological features (Fig. 5.9) differ from the usual types of carcinoma in that extensive dissociation and nuclear pleomorphism are not generally seen. Instead the cardinal feature of the smears is the predominance of compact heaped clusters of monomorphic cells consisting of one cell type. This contrasts with benign clusters which contain a mixture of spindle cells and are usually monolayers. The

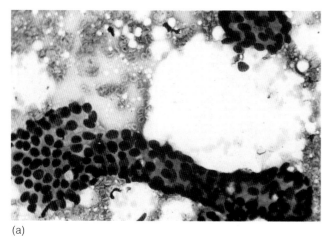

(a)

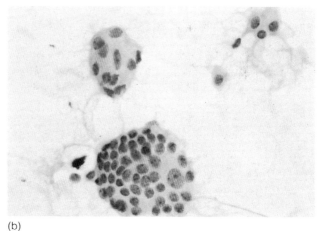

(b)

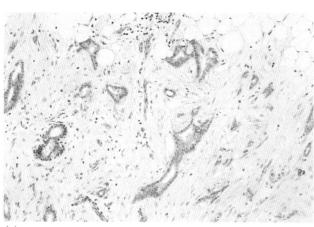

(c)

Figure 5.9 (a) A smear from a case of tubular carcinoma showing tubular glands with a rather well-defined structure. Notice the absence of bare nuclei. The suggestion of two cell types in the clumps could lead to an erroneous diagnosis of a benign lesion (Diff-Quick). (b) Papanicolaou-stained smear from the same case showing abnormal chromatin pattern and some cells with enlarged nuclei (Pap). (c) Tissue section from the same case showing angular tubules infiltrating through desmoplastic stroma (H & E).

clusters of cells are often associated with tubular structures but these are not diagnostic being seen in microglandular adenosis [11] and radial scars [17]. 'Naked' nuclei in pairs may be seen in the background further adding to the difficulty of distinguishing these lesions from benign processes. Many of these tumours are accompanied by cribriform or micropapillary (small cell) carcinoma *in situ* and small heaped-up micropapillary clusters may be seen if the needle has traversed one of the involved *in situ* areas. Atypia may be seen within the cells but in general they are often monomorphic, round and bland in appearance. Some cases do show moderate variation in nuclear size with some flattening of nuclear membranes and hyperchromasia. Nucleoli may also be present. The rare tubulolobular variants of lobular carcinoma [18] often show intracytoplasmic lumina in the cells and tubular carcinoma cells may also contain these.

It is less important to diagnose these tumours unequivocally as malignant than to raise the possibility of malignancy so that the lesion is biopsied. If a positive diagnosis of malignancy can be given then all well and good but it is important not to miss these lesions. Breast screening units which are highly dependent upon the cytology results to avoid benign biopsies should be aware that small spiculate opacities may be difficult to diagnose cytologically and the triple approach [19] should be adhered to. It is important that these lesions are biopsied and not left because of a negative cytology result. Linell *et al.* [20] suggest that tubular carcinoma will become less differentiated with time and that some cases of 'ductal' carcinoma with tubules in the centre of the tumour may start as tubular carcinoma.

Apocrine carcinoma

Apocrine carcinomas are difficult to distinguish from atypical apocrine metaplasia on aspiration cytodiagnosis. The finding of dissociated pleomorphic apocrine cells may not necessarily be diagnostic of apocrine carcinoma but if necrosis is present then one can be more certain of the diagnosis. Some

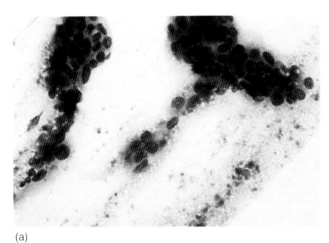

(a)

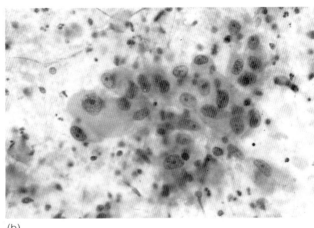

(b)

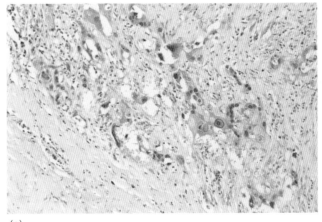

(c)

Figure 5.10 (a) A smear from a case of apocrine carcinoma showing a dirty necrotic background and pleomorphic malignant apocrine cells (compare with Fig. 5.5a) (Diff-Quick). (b) Obvious apocrine features of the malignant cells on Papanicolaou staining from the same case. Note the large single nucleoli (Pap). (c) Tissue section from the same case showing malignant apocrine cells invading the desmoplastic stroma. The whole tumour showed apocrine features (H & E).

authors maintain that if standard criteria are adhered to then a diagnosis of apocrine carcinoma can be confidently made [21]. The standard criteria proposed for pure apocrine carcinoma are many large cells, moderate pleomorphism with few mitoses, mild irregularity of nuclear membranes, a high proportion of dissociated cells, few bare nuclei and necrosis. However, these features are essentially similar to those seen in some rare atypical apocrine proliferations (see *apocrine adenosis*) and it is our view that the diagnosis of apocrine carcinoma should not be made with certainty unless necrotic material or moderate numbers of mitoses are seen (Fig. 5.10).

Squamous carcinoma

Aspirates from squamous carcinoma often contain cystic material and a marked inflammatory component. The malignant squames may on occasions be hard to identify in the inflammatory tissue and cases may turn up as false negatives. Where malignant squames are present in abundance the diagnosis is not a problem but the possibility of metastatic tumour can never be excluded. The majority of squamous carcinomas of the breast occur on the basis of metaplasia within a ductal carcinoma and some lesions may show features of both squamous carcinoma and adenocarcinoma (Fig. 5.11).

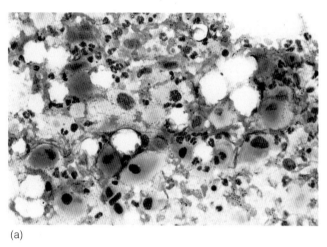

(a)

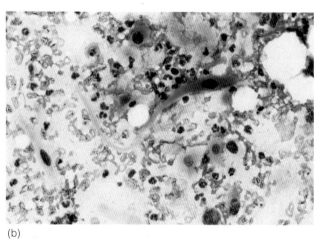

(b)

Figure 5.11 (a) Aspirate of breast mass showing squamous carcinoma. The nuclei are hyperchromatic and occasionally elongated and the cytoplasm stains a bright purple colour with MGG. (b) Another view of squamous carcinoma of the breast. A very long cell is illustrated; others have elongated hyperchromatic nuclei.

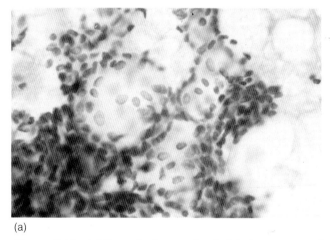

(a)

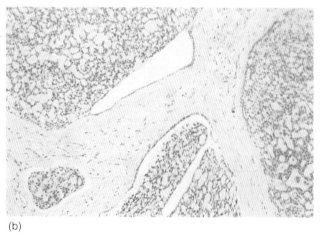

(b)

Figure 5.12 (a) Papanicolaou-stained slide from a case of adenoid cystic carcinoma showing the basement membrane filled pseudocysts. There are apparently two cell types in the clumps and this should not in this instance by regarded as a benign feature. The majority of the cells are of myoepithelial origin (Pap). (b) Tissue section from the same case showing the characteristic biphasic histological pattern of adenoid cystic carcinoma (H & E).

Adenoid cystic carcinoma

The features of adenoid cystic carcinoma of the breast are essentially similar to those seen in the more common salivary gland lesions. The cardinal feature is the finding of eosinophilic hyaline globules of basement membrane material interspersed with the tumour cells. These tumours can appear to have two cell types due to the presence of scanty epithelial tubules interspersed with the myoepithelial cells which make up the majority of the tumour (Fig. 5.12).

Collagenous spherulosis (see earlier) can mimic this tumour and care should be taken to assess nuclear characteristics. Hyperchromasia and moderate nuclear enlargement, together with the clinical presence of a lump are features favouring adenoid cystic carcinoma.

Neuroendocrine carcinoma (argyrophil carcinoma, 'carcinoid tumour')

A number of cases of neuroendocrine carcinoma, some in the male breast, diagnosed on fine needle aspiration have now been reported in the literature. The aspirates are highly cellular and contain monomorphic clusters of small cells of regular size. There is dissociation of similar cells to those in the clusters and the chromatin pattern is often coarsely granular with a small regular nucleolus. The nuclei are somewhat eccentric and some spindling of cells may be seen. Pleomorphism is minimal and bare nuclei are not present. The cells have the cytoplasmic eosinophilia, where the cytoplasm can be evaluated, of neuroendocrine cells. Argyrophilia can be demonstrated on the cytological preparations [22] (Fig. 5.13).

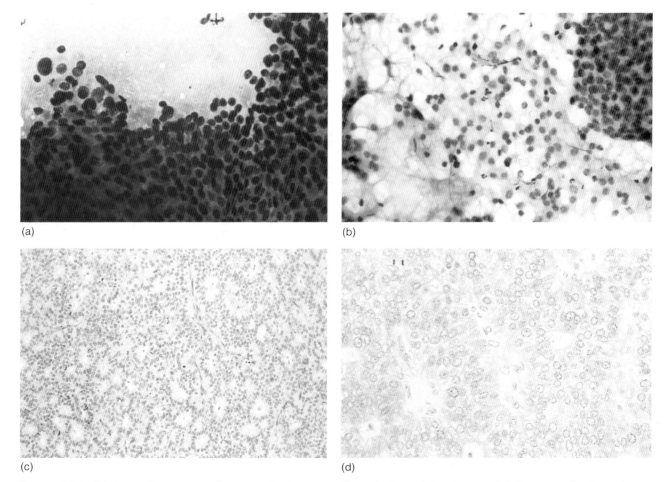

(a)

(b)

(c)

(d)

Figure 5.13　(a) Smear from a case of neuroendocrine carcinoma (argyrophil carcinoma) of the breast showing clumps of cells with nuclear pleomorphism. There is a suggestion of two cell types in the clusters but this should not necessarily be considered as a benign feature (Diff-Quick). (b) The same case showing dissociation of the Papanicolaou-stained smear. (c) Tissue section from the same case showing rosette formation and prominent vascular pattern (H & E). (d) Tissue section from the same case showing positive staining for neuron specific enolase by immunoperoxidase techniques.

MYOEPITHELIAL STROMAL LESIONS

Phyllodes tumours

Phyllodes tumours vary in behaviour from benign cellular fibroadenoma-like lesions with an increased mitotic rate to unequivocal biphasic sarcoma-like lesions. The fine needle aspiration smears (Fig. 5.14) show bare bipolar nuclei similar to those seen in fibroadenoma although they may be somewhat larger. Epithelial clusters are seen and these may appear hyperplastic with heaping-up of cells within them. Stromal fragments are a useful diagnostic feature. These are often seen and are usually much larger than the fragments seen in fibroadenoma. The fragments show an increase in cellularity compared to the fragments seen in fibroadenomas and in some cases nuclear atypia and occasionally mitotic figures may be seen within the stromal cells. Apocrine cells are generally absent. Foam cells, giant cells and occasionally squamous cells may be present. Some cases are difficult to differentiate from fibroadenoma and the diagnosis should be considered in all large lesions over 2 cm which have the cytological characteristics of fibroadenoma [23].

Nodular sclerosing adenosis

Nodular sclerosing adenosis, otherwise known as 'adenosis tumour', has in the past caused problems in 'frozen' section histological diagnosis and is now being sampled by fine needle aspiration. According to the literature the cytological diagnosis is unlike carcinoma [24], the lesion giving a cellular appearance with the classical features of benignity. Uniform clusters of ductal cells, numerous bipolar bare nuclei and stromal fragments are seen. Cytologically, although the lesion is characteristically shown to be benign, a definitive diagnosis of nodular sclerosing adenosis cannot be made.

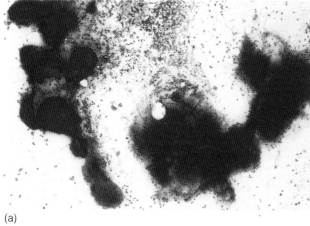

(a)

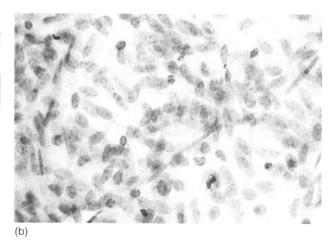

(b)

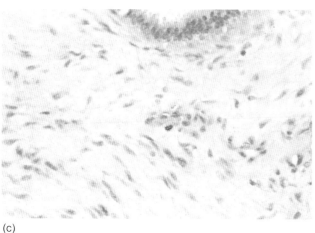

(c)

Figure 5.14 (a) Smear from a case of phyllodes tumour showing metachromatic stromal tissue and benign appearing compact epithelial clusters (Diff-Quick). (b) Hypercellular stroma from the same case showing nuclear pleomorphism and a mitotic figure (Pap). (c) Tissue section from the same case showing stromal cellularity and mitosis (H & E).

Adenomyoepithelioma

Adenomyoepithelioma is a rather ill-defined entity [25] which seems to encompass two main types of lesion. There are benign-appearing lesions which resemble adenomas but which have a proliferative myoepithelial component. In these tumours there is little or no atypia in either the stromal or epithelial components. Fine needle aspiration [26] of these can be difficult (Fig. 5.15). The smears are cellular and show large three-dimensional clusters of epithelial cells, rather than the flat monolayers usually seen in benign lesions. An apparent dissociation of some moderately sized cells with eosinophilic nucleoli is seen and these form small clusters or even small tubules. The clue to the benign diagnosis is the moderate numbers of bare nuclei in the background. The lesion can be misinterpreted as being a small cell carcinoma of lobular type within an area of hyperplastic cystic change. Over-diagnosis should be avoided by recognizing the bare nuclei and resisting the temptation to call smears with abundant bare nuclei malignant.

The other type of adenomyoepithelial lesion is rarer and has a rather pleomorphic myoepithelial component overgrowing the epithelial elements. Mitoses may be present and histologically sheets of clears cells are seen. Some of these tumours have been reported to metastasize to axillary nodes. They should be regarded as tumours of low grade malignant potential. Specific cytodiagnosis is not possible.

Pleomorphic adenoma

Pleomorphic adenoma (Fig. 5.16) is histologically similar to those cases seen in the salivary gland. They are really variants of adenomyoepitheliomas where the myoepithelial component has produced the characteristic chrondromyxoid stroma.

The fine needle aspiration appearances may be very cellular and consist generally of clumps of cells of epithelial appearance set within metachromatic myxoid material on Giemsa staining. There are dissociated cells with cytoplasm but also bare nuclei are present. The myxoid material is highly characteristic and should not be mistaken for the mucus of a mucinous carcinoma [27].

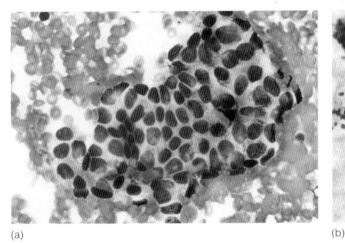
(a)

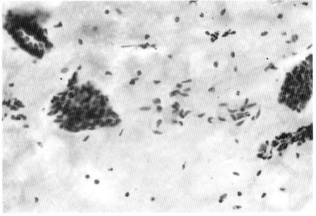
(b)

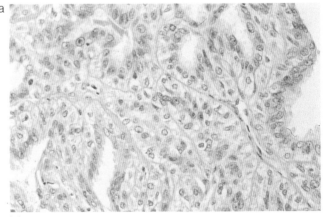
(c)

Figure 5.15 (a) Smear from a case of adenomyoepithelioma of the breast. Note the pleomorhism but also the peripheral spindle cells and the suggestion of two cell types (Diff-Quick). (b) The same case on the Papanicolaou stain showing bare nuclei, tubule formation and some stromal cells. (c) Tissue section from the resected specimen showing tubular epithelial structures and myoepithelial proliferation (H & E).

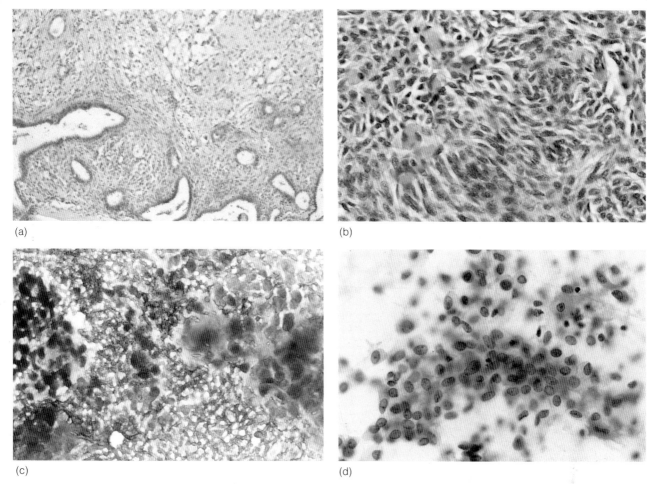

(a)

(b)

(c)

(d)

Figure 5.16 (a) Low-power photomicrograph of the histology of a pleomorphic adenoma of the breast. Epithelial clefts are seen from which myoepithelial cells stream, some of which differentiate into cartilage at the bottom left-hand corner. (b) High-power view of the histology showing spindle-shaped myoepithelial cells. (c) Low-power view of the aspirate showing purple-staining stroma and loose aggregates of large cells (Giemsa). (d) High-power Papanicolaou-stained cytospin preparation showing cells similar to those seen in (b).

SOFT TISSUE LESIONS

Fibromatosis and nodular fasciitis

Fibromatosis may present clinically as an irregular hard, enlarging mass mimicking carcinoma. The mammographic features may also resemble those of a carcinoma. It usually produces a poorly cellular aspirate [28] which is not surprising considering its histological appearance of bands of infiltrating spindly fibrous cells (Fig. 5.17).

A similar condition with almost identical clinical features is nodular fasciitis. The aspirate will be sparsely cellular with some epithelial cells, macrophages, fibroblasts and lymphocytes present [29].

Schwannoma

The cytological features of schwannoma occurring in the breast were described by Fisher *et al.* in an article in 1990 [30]. The smears showed cellular clusters of spindle cells with no signficant atypia. They note that the features were those mainly of Antoni A areas. No breast epithelium was present.

Granular cell tumour

Granular cell tumour is occasionally found in the breast. The features in needle aspirates are the presence of moderate numbers of dissociated foamy cells with a clear or light-pink cytoplasm on Papanicolaou stains and a light-blue cytoplasm on May–Grünwald Giemsa staining (Fig. 5.18). Nuclei may be variable but do not have an abnormal chromatin pattern in general and the nuclear-cytoplasmic ratio is low. The nuclei are generally stated to stain poorly in aspirate specimens [31]. Once the diagnosis is remembered then the potential for false positive diagnosis is minimized but occasional cases can be a little pleomorphic and it is as well to remember that they may appear malignant clinically and radiologically.

Lymphoma

Lymphoma of the breast is an unusual finding which most commonly occurs in association with known generalized lymphoma and hence usually presents no diagnostic problem. Some cases however, are either primary breast lymphoma or the first presentation of more generalized disease. The majority of the lesions are B-cell non-Hodgkin's lymphoma although occasional reports of T-cell lymphoma have appeared [32]. The cytology of lymphoma may present a diagnostic problem in differentiating the malignant cells from carcinoma. In general lymphoma cells show complete or almost complete dissociation with none of the clusters usually seen in carcinoma (Fig. 5.19). One type of small cell carcinoma does produce almost complete dissociation of rather plasmacytic-appearing cells, but it should be remembered that lymphomas are usually high grade and plasmacytic or lymphoplasmacytoid variants in the breast are exceedingly rare. In cases of doubt epithelial and lymphoid markers can be applied to cytological smears.

Differentiating between carcinoma and lymphoma in needle aspirates is very important as segmental excision or mastectomy are inappropriate treatments for lymphoma. Chloroma has also been diagnosed by needle aspiration cytodiagnosis [33].

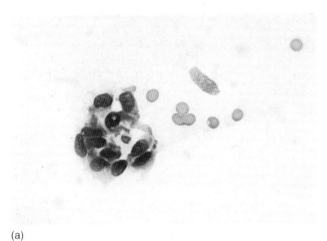

(a)

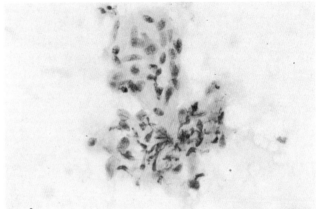

(b)

Figure 5.17 (a) Aspirate from a case of fibromatosis showing scanty small stromal cells with no significant pleomorphism (Diff-Quick). (b) The same case on the Papanicolaou stain. There is a little crushing artefact to the cells in the lower part of the field. (c) Histological section from the same case showing dense, poorly cellular fibrous tissue at the lower left, infiltrating between normal breast lobules (H & E).

(c)

Hamartoma

Hamartoma may be palpable or detected by mammography which can be diagnostic. The mammographic appearance is that of a fairly well-defined mass showing mixed densities relating to the fat and stromal elements. The aspirate contains only non-specific features such as clusters of fat cells, stromal fragments and scanty benign epithelial cells. It is indistinguishable cytologically from normal breast tissue.

Haemangiosarcoma/lymphangiosarcoma

Sarcomas of the breast are rare lesions but one of the more common is the angiosarcoma. This tumour may occur in the breast *de novo* but may also occur after radiotherapy and in chronic lymphoedema of the arm (Stewart–Trieves syndrome).

The range of histological appearance is wide varying from well-differentiated tumours showing bland vascular channels to frankly sarcomatous spindle-cell tumours. The cytological appearances

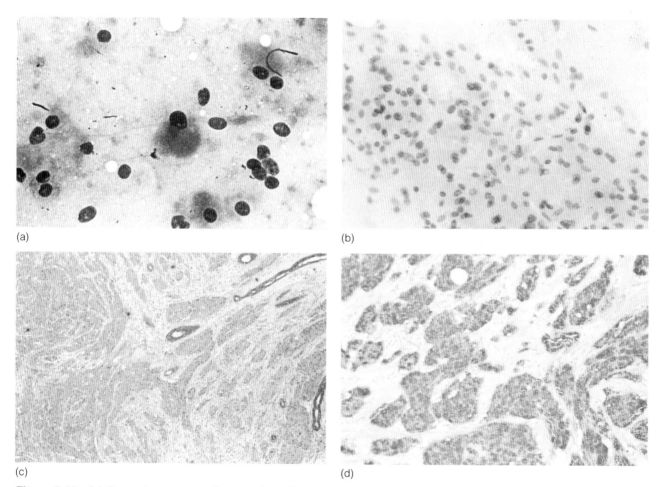

(a)

(b)

(c)

(d)

Figure 5.18 (a) Smear from a case of a granular cell tumour of the breast showing a rather dirty background and mildly pleomorphic cells with a large amount of granular cytoplasm. Some of the nuclei are stripped of cytoplasm but are not the normal bare nuclei found in benign aspirates (Giemsa). Cytology kindly provided courtesy of Dr J. McKenzie and Dr J. Dalrymple, St Margaret's Hospital, Epping. (b) Papanicolaou-stained smear from the same case showing the granular nature of the cell cytoplasm. (c) Tissue section from the same case showing normal ducts surrounded by granular eosinophilic cells (H & E). Histology sections of the same case kindly provided by Dr A. Ahmed, Chelmsford Hospital. (d) Tissue section stained for S100 protein by the immunoperoxidase technique to show the positive tumour cells.

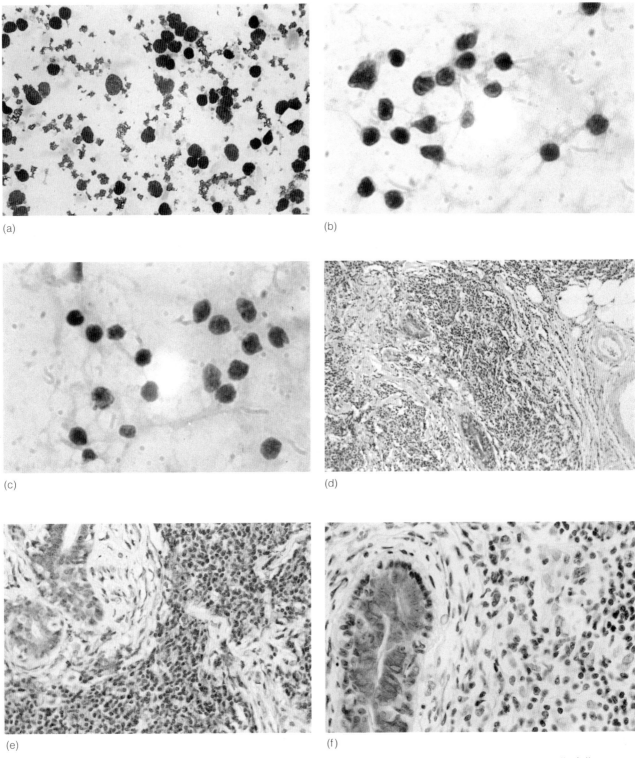

(a)

(b)

(c)

(d)

(e)

(f)

Figure 5.19 (a) Aspirate of a breast lymphoma showing pleomorphic lymphoid cells with total dissociation. Blasts and smaller lymphocytes can be seen. The appearances are those of a low-grade centrocytic–centroblastic lymphoma (Diff-Quick). (b) Immunoperoxidase for a B-cell marker (L26) on a direct methanol-fixed smear in the same case showing cytoplasmic positivity (oil immersion). (c) Immunoperoxidase for a T-cell marker (CD3) showing negative cytoplasm around the malignant cells (oil immersion). (d) Tissue section from the same case showing lymphomatous infiltration around normal breast ducts (H & E). (e) L26 immunoperoxidase for B-cells on a frozen section of the same case showing the lymphoid cells to be positive. (f) CAM 5.2 immunoperoxidase for epithelial cells from the same case showing a positive duct with surrounding negative lymphoma cells.

reflect this (Fig. 5.20). Reports of the cytology of well-differentiated angiosarcomas of the breast [34] and other sites [35] suggest the smears are hypocellular with small loose groups of tumour cells showing moderate variation in size, nuclear grooves, complex nuclear infoldings and nuclear moulding. Spindle cells are uncommon in these tumours though occasionally seen. Some tumours show papillary clusters which can be mistaken for DCIS.

Poorly differentiated angiosarcomas show malignant spindle cells and large amounts of blood. They are not always distinguishable from other sarcomas or poorly differentiated spindle cell carcinomas on morphology alone and Factor VIII immunostaining may be necessary for differentiation.

Stromal sarcoma

Sarcomas of the breast can be typed according to the various patterns encountered elsewhere in the body. Berg *et al.* [36] coined the term 'stromal sarcoma' for cases of sarcoma within the breast but it may be more appropriate however to restrict the term to

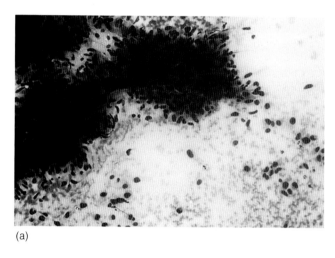

(a)

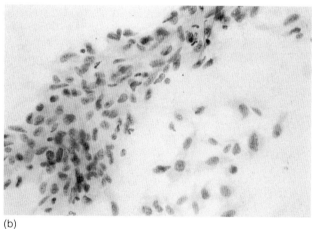

(b)

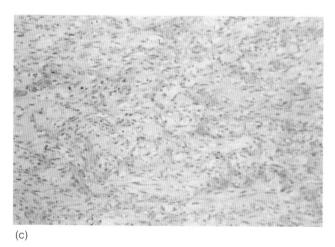

(c)

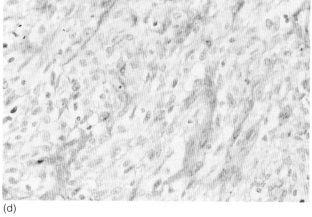

(d)

Figure 5.20 (a) Smear from a case of poorly differentiated angiosarcoma showing clumps of malignant spindle cells with dissociation (Diff-Quick). (b) Papanicolaou-stained smear from the same case. (c) Tissue section from the same case showing poorly formed vascular structures within the tumour (H & E). (d) Factor VIII immunoperoxidase on the tumour cells showing positivity indicating origin from endothelium.

tumours of lobular connective tissue as described by Rupp *et al.* [37]. These tumours are similar to malignant phyllodes tumours but lack the epithelial component. Fine needle aspiration shows atypical spindle cells, singly or in small clusters. It is not however usually profitable to attempt to type these tumours on fine needle aspiration as the absence of an epithelial component can only be proven on histological examination (Fig. 5.21).

Haemangiopericytoma

Fine needle aspiration of this rare lesion of the breast has been described [38] as showing vascular capillaries which stain for Factor VIII surrounded by 'knob-like' formations of spindle-to-oval cells which stain for vimentin only. These are the pericytes which form the tumour. For practical purposes a diagnosis of 'spindle cell neoplasm' may be all that is necessary in reporting fine needle aspiration specimens from such lesions and biopsy of these rare conditions will often be required for definitive typing.

REFERENCES

1. Rosen, P. P. and Kimmel, M. (1990) Juvenile papillomatosis of breast: A follow-up study of 41 patients having biopsies before 1979. *Am. J. Clin. Pathol.* **93**, 599–603.
2. Rosen, P. P., Holmes, G., Lesser, M. L. *et al.* (1985) Juvenile papillomatosis and breast carcinoma. *Cancer*, **55**(6), 1345–52.
3. Azzopardi, J. G. and Salm, R. (1984) Ductal adenoma of the breast: A lesion which can mimic carcinoma. *J. Pathol.*, **144**, 15–23.
4. Taylor, H. B. and Robertson, A. G. (1965) Adenomas of the nipple. *Cancer*, **18**, 995–1002.
5. Stormby, N. and Bondeson, L. (1984) Adenoma of the nipple; an unusual diagnosis in aspiration cytology. *Acta Cytol.* **28**, 729–32.
6. Martin-Bates, E., Krausz, T. and Phillips, I. (1990) Evaluation of fine needle aspiration of the male breast for the diagnosis of gynaecomastia. *Cytopathology*, **1**, 79–85.
7. Chang, A. R. (1990) Fine needle aspiration cytology in a case of florid gynaecomastia. *Cytopathology*, **1**, 357–61.

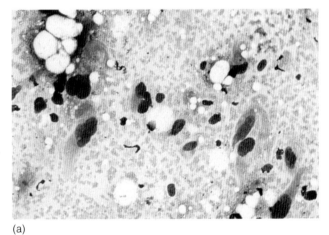

(a)

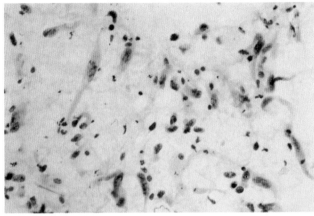

(b)

Figure 5.21 (a) Malignant spindle cells in a smear from a case of stromal sarcoma of the breast (Diff-Quick). (b) Papanicolaou-stained smear from the same case. (c) Tissue section from the same case showing a highly malignant sarcoma invading the breast tissue (H & E). Histology courtesy of Dr G. Farrer-Brown, London.

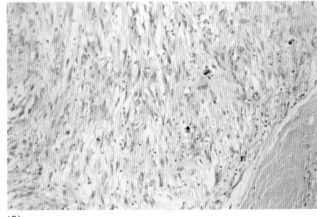

(c)

8. Pinedo, F., Vargas, J., de Agustín, P. *et al.* (1991) Epithelial atypia in gynecomastia induced by chemotherapeutic drugs: A possible pitfall in fine needle aspiration biopsy. *Acta Cytol.* **35**, 229–33.

9. Simpson, J. F., Page, D. L. and Dupont, W. D. (1990) Apocrine adenosis – a mimic of mammary carcinoma. *Surg. Pathol.*, **3**, 289–99.

10. Makunura, C. M., Curling, O. M., Yeomans, P. *et al.* (1994) Apocrine adenosis within a radial scar: A false positive diagnosis for carcinoma of the breast. *Cytopathology* **5**, 123–8.

11. Evans, A. T. and Hussein, K. A. H. (1990) A microglandular adenosis-like lesion simulating tubular adenocarcinoma of the breast. A case report with cytological and histological appearances. *Cytopathology*, **1**, 311–6.

12. Wells, C. A., Wells, C. W., Yeomans, P. *et al.* (1990) Spherical connective tissue inclusions in epithelial hyperplasia of the breast ('collagenous spherulosis') *J. Clin. Pathol.* **43**, 905–8.

13. Tyler, X. and Coghill, S. B. (1991) Fine needle aspiration cytology of collagenous spherulosis of the breast. *Cytopathology*, **2**, 159–62.

14. Dupont, W. and Page, D. L. (1985) Risk factors for breast cancer in women with proliferative disease. *N. Engl. J. Med.* **312**, 146–51.

15. Salhany, K. E. and Page, D. L. (1989) Fine-needle aspiration of mammary lobular carcinoma *in situ* and atypical lobular hyperplasia. *Am. J. Clin. Pathol.* **92**(1), 22–6.

16. Abendroth, C. S., Wang, H. H. and Ducatman, B. S. (1991) Comparative features of carcinoma *in situ* and atypical ductal hyperplasia of the breast on fine needle aspiration biopsy specimens. *Am. J. Clin. Pathol.* **96**, 654–9,

17. Bondeson, L. and Lindholm, K. (1990) Aspiration cytology of tubular breast carcinoma. *Acta Cytol.* **34**(1), 15–20.

18. Fisher, E. R., Gregorio, R. M., Redmond, C. and Fisher, B. (1977) Tubulolobular invasive breast cancer: a variant of lobular invasive cancer. *Human Pathol.* **8**, 679–83.

19. Lamb, J., Anderson, T. J., Dixon, M. J. and Levack, P. (1987) Role of fine needle aspiration cytology in breast cancer screening. *J. Clin. Pathol.* **40**, 705–9.

20. Linell, F., Ljungberg, O. and Andersson, I. (1980) Breast carcinoma: Aspects of early stages, progression and related problems. *Acta Pathol. Microbiol. Scand.* (suppl) **227A**, 1–233.

21. Gupta, R. K., McHutchison, A. G. R., Simpson, J. S. and Dowle, C. S. (1992) Fine needle aspiration cytodiagnosis of apocrine carcinoma of the breast. *Cytopathology*, **3**, 321–6.

22. Ravinsky, E. and Cavers, D. J. (1985) Cytology of argyrophilic carcinoma of the breast. *Acta Cytol.* **29**, 1–6.

23. Simu, U., Moretti, D., Iacconi, P. *et al.* (1988) Fine needle aspiration cytopathology of phyllodes tumor; differential diagnosis with fibroadenoma. *Acta Cytol.* **32**, 63–6.

24. Silverman, J. F., Dabbs, D. J. and Falbert, C. F. (1989) Fine needle aspiration cytology of adenosis tumor of the breast with immunocytochemical and ultrastructure observations. *Acta Cytol.* **33**, 181–7.

25. Loose, J. H., Patchefsky, A. S., Hollander, I. J. *et al.* (1992) Adenomyoepithelioma of the breast: a spectrum of biologic behavior. *Am. J. Surg. Pathol.* **16**, 868–76.

26. Vielh, P., Thiery, J. P. and Validire, P. (1993) Adenomyoepithelioma of the breast: Fine needle sampling with histologic, immunohistologic, and electron microscopic analysis. *Diag. Cytopath.* **9**, 188–93.

27. Chen, K. T. K. (1990) Pleomorphic adenoma of the breast. *Am. J. Clin. Pathol.* **93**, 792–4.

28. Pettinato, G., Manivel, J. C., Petrella, G. and Jassim, A. D. (1991) Fine needle aspiration cytology, immunocytochemistry and electron microscopy of fibromatosis of the breast: Report of two cases. *Acta Cytol.* **35**, 403–8.

29. Fritsches, H. G. and Muller, E. A. (1983) Pseudosarcomatous fasciitis of the breast. Cytologic and histologic features. *Acta Cytol.* **27**, 73–5.

30. Fisher, P. E., Esterbrook, A. and Gohen, M. B. (1990) Fine needle aspiration biopsy of intramammary neurilemmoma. *Acta Cytol.* **34**, 35–7.

31. Löwhagen, T. and Rubio, C. A. (1977) The cytology of the granular cell myoblastoma of the breast. Report of a case. *Acta Cytol.* **21**, 314–5.

32. Pettinato, G., Manivel, J. C., Petrella, G. and De Chiara, A. (1991) Primary multilobated T-cell lymphoma of the breast diagnosed by fine needle aspiration cytology and immunocytochemistry. *Acta Cytol.* **35**, 294–9.

33. Pettinato, G., De Ghiara, A., Insabato, L. and De Renzo, A. (1988) Fine needle aspiration biopsy of a granulocytic sarcoma (chloroma) of the breast. *Acta Cytol.* **32**, 67–73.

34. Masin, M. and Masin. F. (1978) Cytology of angiosarcoma of the breast: a case report. *Acta Cytol.* **22**, 162–4.

35. Abele, J. and Miller, T. (1982) Cytology of well-differentiated and poorly differentiated hemangiosarcoma in fine needle aspirates. *Acta Cytol.* **26**, 341–8.

36. Berg, J. W., DeCrosse, J. J., Fracchia, A. A. and Farrow, J. (1962) Stromal sarcomas of the breast. A unified approach to connective tissue sarcomas other than cystosarcoma phyllodes. *Cancer*, **15**, 418–24.

37. Rupp, M., Hafiz, M. A., Khalluf, E. and Sutula, M. (1988) Fine needle aspiration in stromal sarcoma of the breast; light and electron microscopic findings with histologic correlation. *Acta Cytol.* **32**, 72–4.

38. Jiménez-Ayala, M., Díez-Nau, M. D., Larrad, A. *et al.* (1991) Hemangiopericytoma in a male breast: Report of a case with cytologic, histologic and immunochemical studies. *Acta Cytol.* **35**, 234–8.

6. Nipple smears

Grace McKee

INTRODUCTION

The nipple, surrounded by the areola, is covered by keratinized stratified squamous epithelium. Its surface contains the openings of fifteen to twenty lactiferous ducts. These ducts are lined by squamous epithelium near the surface of the nipple and by cuboidal epithelium elsewhere.

The examination of nipple smears and discharge specimens can be of diagnostic value in local and systemic breast disease. However, nipple discharge can be physiological in girls at puberty and when lactation continues after breast feeding has ceased. Nipple secretion may be due to mechanical factors such as compression of the breast at mammography, and is seen as a side effect of taking some drugs such as phenothiazines and oral contraceptives. Bilateral serous nipple discharge may be symptomatic of a pituitary tumour [1] especially in patients with amenorrhoea and raised prolactin levels.

Unilateral nipple discharge usually relates to local disease and the evidence of origin from a single lactiferous duct should be obtained by careful inspection. Blood-stained, or discoloured fluid has an association with underlying tumour but not all bloody discharges indicate a neoplasm, and clear fluid should not be discounted as an innocent event. The presence of blood can be confirmed by Hemastix testing.

In an analysis of 176 patients having microdochectomy [2] for blood-stained or persistent discharge, 15 (9%) had carcinoma, 78 (44%) had an intraduct papilloma and the rest a range of abnormalities including duct ectasia, fibrocystic change, inflammation, epitheliosis and hyperplasia. The percentage with bloody discharge was only slightly higher (59%) in the neoplastic group compared to the remainder (56%).

The preparation of nipple discharge smears for cytological examination is simplicity itself. A clean glass slide is labelled in pencil on the frosted end with the patient's name. The nipple is then touched gently with the centre of the slide and the resulting smear is either rapidly fixed in alcohol or air-dried. Secretion can be encouraged by compressing the breast, and several smears prepared. Gentleness and speed produce the best results. Radiographers are well placed to observe any nipple secretion produced during mammography and can be instructed on how to make good quality smears for cytological assessment.

Another method of obtaining smears is by using breast pumps or suction devices [3]. The devices have varied but generally consist of a transparent circular airtight chamber connected to a syringe or pump to create a vacuum which sucks out nipple fluid. Although both *in situ* and infiltrating carcinoma can be detected by this method [4], in asymptomatic women it was found to be insufficiently sensitive for screening purposes. In a prospective study [5] using this method, covering a period of 18 years, it was shown that the demonstration of

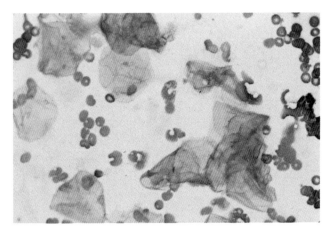

Figure 6.1 Cytology of a normal nipple scrape. In a wet-fixed smear squamous cells stain a refractile orange as they are keratinized. They have no nuclei and their cytoplasm is often folded upon itself (Pap).

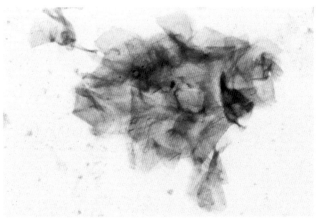

Figure 6.2 Cytology of a normal nipple scrape. In an air-dried smear squames appear as azure blue, often folded cells with no nuclei. These cells have been scraped off the surface of keratinized squamous epithelium (MGG).

cellular hyperplasia could antedate the development of carcinoma.

A smear taken from a normal healthy nipple shows only anucleate keratinized squames from the skin surface. These are seen on a wet-fixed, Papanicolaou-stained smear as large flat or folded orange staining cells without nuclei (Fig. 6.1). In an air-dried smear which has been stained using the May–Grünwald Giemsa method, keratinized anucleate squames stain a characteristic shade of azure blue (Fig. 6.2).

LACTATION

The microscopic examination of milk shows a few epithelial cells but mainly macrophages in a proteinaceous fluid in which fat is present in the form of small empty vacuoles (Figs 6.3 and 6.4). In air-dried smears the fat can be demonstrated using Oil red O but in wet-fixed smears it is dispersed by the alcohol. The macrophages show a foamy appearance (Figs 6.5 and 6.6) which consists of finely vacuolated cytoplasm and they often have indistinct cell bor-

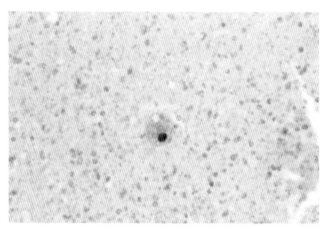

Figure 6.3 Cytology of a milk secretion smear. A fluid background which is composed of proteinaceous and lipid-rich material and a single foamy macrophage is seen (Pap).

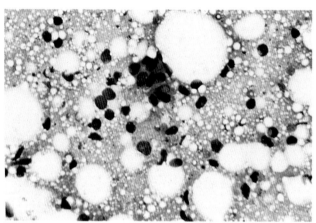

Figure 6.4 Cytology of a milk secretion smear. Note the more obvious bubbly, lipid-rich proteinaceous material in the background of this air-dried smear. A few benign epithelial cells and some foamy macrophages are present (MGG).

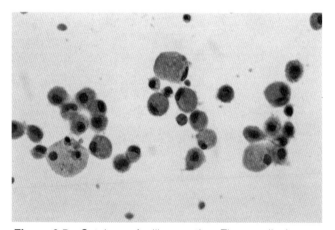

Figure 6.5 Cytology of milk secretion. These cells, known as foamy macrophages or foam cells have abundant cytoplasm, eccentric, sharply defined nuclei and conspicuous nucleoli. The cell size varies greatly (Pap).

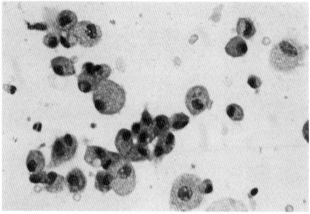

Figure 6.6 Cytology of milk secretion. This air-dried smear shows macrophages with abundant foamy cytoplasm and eccentric nuclei (MGG).

ders. The nucleus is eccentric and generally has a sharp outline and a conspicuous nucleolus. The cells may be binucleated or even multinucleated.

GALACTOCOELE

A galactocoele is the accumulation of milk in ducts below the nipple after termination of lactation causing the dilation of ducts and cyst formation, and occasionally a palpable lump in the breast containing inspissated milk. The examination of a nipple secretion gives a clue to the diagnosis as the smears show a bubbly background of lipid-filled material and benign epithelial cells showing secretory changes (Fig. 6.7).

FIBROCYSTIC CHANGE

The term fibrocystic change has been used to denote benign proliferative and degenerative changes of the breast, otherwise known as benign mastopathy, and more recently as Aberration of Normal Development and Involution (ANDI) (see Chapter 2). Fibrocystic change includes a wide range of histological patterns such as cystic changes, adenosis, apocrine metaplasia, epitheliosis, papillomatosis and epithelial hyperplasia. Nipple discharge in this condition occurs when a subareolar cyst has formed which connects to a lactiferous duct. Nipple smears usually contain foamy macrophages and a few benign ductal cells in a proteinaceous background [6].

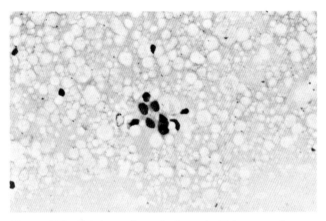

Figure 6.7 Cytology of a galactocoele. This smear from a galactocoele shows a similar bubbly background to that of milk secretion with a few benign cells. No foamy macrophages are noted in this field (Pap).

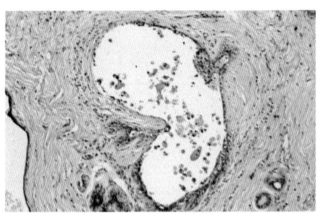

Figure 6.8 Histology of periductal inflammation. In this section there is a dilated duct filled with foamy macrophages. The wall of the duct shows a patchy chronic inflammatory cell infiltrate (H & E).

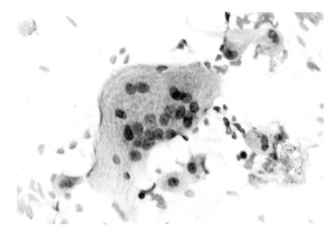

Figure 6.9 Cytology of nipple discharge in duct ectasia. This wet-fixed smear shows a multinucleated giant histiocyte (macrophage) which seems to be continuous with a smaller foamy macrophage. Other foamy macrophages are visible in the background (Pap).

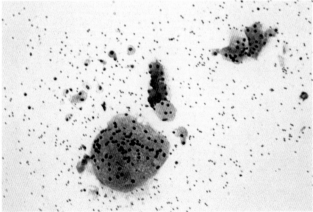

Figure 6.10 Cytology of nipple discharge in duct ectasia. The air-dried smear shows a large multinucleated macrophage which has the same foamy cytoplasm and nuclei that are seen in the nearby foamy macrophages (MGG).

DUCT ECTASIA

Duct ectasia is a condition seen usually in perimenopausal women in which there is dilation of the large ducts below the nipple to form a mass and associated stromal inflammation. This is usually a chronic process with fibrosis which can cause contraction and nipple inversion so that a clinical diagnosis of carcinoma is sometimes made. The clinical intraluminal secretion consists of concentrated proteinaceous and fatty material, and the epithelium appears attenuated. The periductal inflammation, which is presumably due to the cyst contents leaking intermittently into the surrounding tissue, often consists largely of plasma cells (Fig. 6.8) with fewer lymphocytes and polymorphs.

Nipple discharge related to duct ectasia is usually serous but may be haemorrhagic [2]. The smears show a granular proteinaceous background with scattered foamy macrophages. There are occasionally multinucleated giant histiocytes present which appear to be formed by the union of small foamy macrophages (Figs 6.9 and 6.10). They resemble foreign body giant cells with nuclei randomly scattered within the cytoplasm. Small clusters of ductal cells have been reported in nipple discharge specimens associated with duct ectasia [6] but in the author's experience, and in that of others, epithelial cells are rarely seen [7]. Some foamy macrophages are believed to originate from epithelial cells [8], but some foam cells are true macrophages.

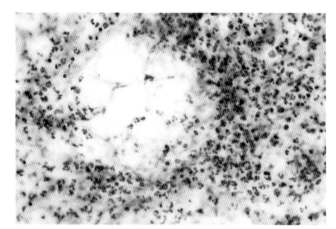

Figure 6.11 Cytology of nipple discharge in mastitis. Numerous polymorphs and scattered foamy macrophages are seen. No epithelial cells are evident (Pap).

ACUTE INFLAMMATION

In conditions such as acute mastitis located near the nipple, there is sometimes a nipple discharge which consists of numerous polymorphs and a few macrophages and multinucleated histiocytes with background debris (Fig. 6.11). Epithelial cells are not usually seen.

DUCT PAPILLOMA

This common benign neoplasm arises from both large and small ducts. Patients present with a unilateral nipple discharge which is usually serous but may be blood-stained. More than one papilloma may be present involving several ducts and it may be palpable if situated beneath the areola. It has been reported in a male following phenothiazine therapy [9]. Symptomatic duct papillomas are rarely visible on a mammogram but screening may show suspicious mammographic findings that prompt biopsy and reveal a papilloma (Figs 6.12 and 6.13). Histologically a duct papilloma shows a papillary growth pattern with a central fibrovascular core and feathery or frond-like branches covered by cuboidal epithelial cells resting on a layer of myoepithelial cells (Fig. 6.14).

The nipple smear often contains both fresh and altered blood with many scattered foamy macrophages. When altered blood is present, indicative of previous haemorrhage into the affected duct, many siderophages are usually present. Haemosiderin appears as yellowish-brown granules in the cytoplasm of the macrophage in wet-fixed smears stained by the Papanicolaou method (Fig. 6.15). In air-dried smears stained with the May–Grünwald Giemsa stain, haemosiderin stains dark blue (Fig. 6.16). The hallmark of a duct papilloma is the presence of papillary clusters of small cohesive benign ductal cells. The clusters themselves are usually small and the cells show variation from bland ductal cells to slightly enlarged cells with visible nucleoli (Figs 6.17 and 6.18). Occasionally the cells show a 'cupping' arrangement (Fig. 6.19). Apocrine cells may be seen infrequently.

PAPILLARY CARCINOMA

Patients with papillary-type mammary carcinoma often present with a nipple discharge which is usually blood-stained. It is much less common than duct papilloma amounting to about 16 per cent of

Figure 6.12 Mammogram of duct papilloma. There is a group of variable-shaped microcalcification particles associated with an ill-defined lobulated mass. These indeterminate findings prompted biopsy which revealed a duct papilloma (Courtesy of Dr Julie Cooke).

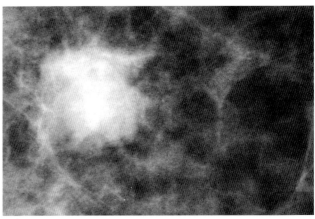

Figure 6.13 Mammogram of duct papilloma. There is an ill-defined mass with a hazy margin. The mammographic findings are suspicious for malignancy and biopsy was carried out. The histology showed a benign duct papilloma (Courtesy of Dr Julie Cooke).

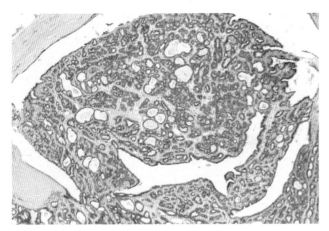

Figure 6.14 Histology of duct papilloma. The section shows papillary structures with connective tissue cores covered by two layers of cells – benign epithelial cells and myoepithelial cells (H & E).

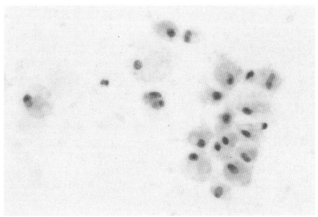

Figure 6.15 Cytology of duct papilloma. This wet-fixed nipple discharge smear shows many foamy macrophages. The one in the centre of the field contains intracytoplasmic yellowish-brown pigment granules which are haemosiderin (Pap).

Figure 6.16 Cytology of duct papilloma. The foamy macrophages seen in this air-dried nipple discharge smear contain heavy clumps of dark-blue pigment within their cytoplasm. This is haemosiderin. The surrounding red cells are not intact but have started to disintegrate and represent altered blood (MGG).

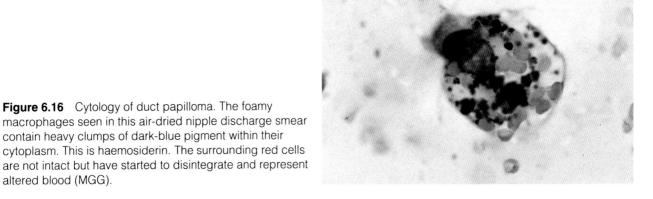

cases of papillary lesions presenting with single duct nipple discharge. The cytological distinction between papilloma and papillary carcinoma relies on cytological features indicating malignancy that include a high nuclear-cytoplasmic ratio, nuclear atypia and large cells. Quite often the pathologist can only be suspicious of a neoplasm and in the paper by Fung *et al.* [2] in which patients with single duct nipple discharge were investigated, those with malignant and suspicious cytology were grouped together. Ten of 15 cases of carcinoma showed abnormal cytology and three out of 61 patients with a solitary papilloma were also thought to be abnormal. Mammography as an aid to diagnosis in this series was found to be unreliable.

Papillary carcinoma is found in rather older women than conventional carcinoma and a palpable mass is usually present. Many are cystic and some involve a pyramidal-shaped area centering on the areola. The histological diagnosis includes consideration of the pattern of growth although this is thought to be less important than the cytology. The

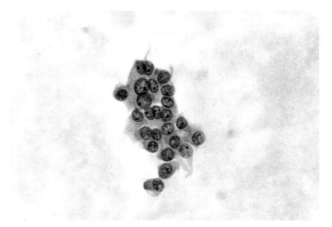

Figure 6.17 Cytology of duct papilloma. This field shows a cluster of fairly uniform cells with rounded nuclei and visible nucleoli representing exfoliated cells from a duct papilloma. A mild degree of atypia may be seen in some cases, for example the prominent granular chromatin noted in these cells (Pap).

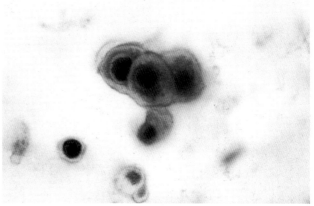

Figure 6.19 Cytology of duct papilloma. In this nipple discharge smear there is a group of slightly enlarged epithelial cells showing 'cupping'. A certain degree of atypia is permitted in duct papillomas but careful examination is essential to exclude carcinoma (Pap). (See Fig. 6.24 for comparison).

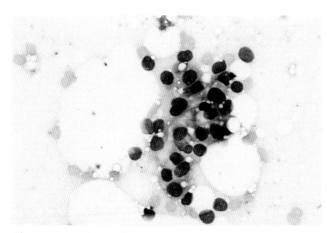

Figure 6.18 Cytology of duct papilloma. This air-dried nipple discharge smear shows a cluster of benign ductal cells with nuclei about the same size as the adjacent erythrocytes. The cell dissociation is artefactual (MGG).

carcinoma is formed by branching papillary fronds protruding into a central cavity. The prognosis is generally better than that of ductal carcinoma NOS as a consequence of their exophytic intracystic growth pattern.

CARCINOMA OF THE BREAST INCLUDING DCIS

Carcinoma occurring in close proximity to the nipple is more likely to exfoliate cells which appear in nipple secretions than neoplasms occurring at other sites in the breast. In some instances nipple discharge may be the first symptom noted by the patient. This may be accompanied by a normal mammogram. In some cases mammography shows the typical features of calcification associated with *in situ* ductal carcinoma (Fig. 6.22). Clinically there may

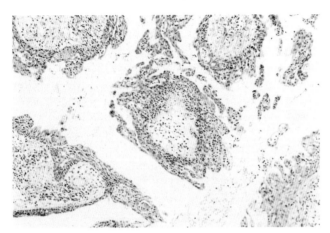

Figure 6.20 Histology of nipple adenoma. The section shows papillary fronds composed of delicate vascular connective tissue cores covered by epithelial cells and myoepithelial cells. No evidence of malignancy is seen (H & E).

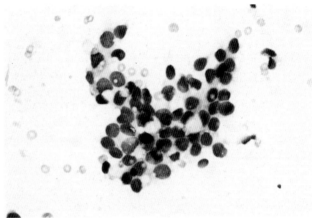

Figure 6.21 Cytology of nipple adenoma. This wet-fixed nipple discharge smear shows a cluster of mildly pleomorphic epithelial cells which are loosely cohesive. There are no features of malignancy (MGG).

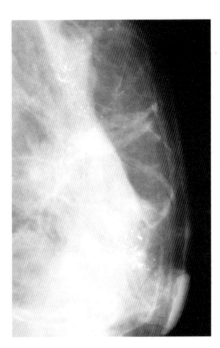

Figure 6.22 Mammogram showing malignant calcification. This shows two separate clusters of malignant-type calcification. The individual particles show marked variation in their size, shape and density. Some are linear within ducts, others are branching, showing the outline of duct bifurcations. These features are typical of comedo-type ductal carcinoma *in situ*. Although the majority of cases are impalpable and symptom-free, those situated near the nipple may present with a blood-stained nipple discharge (Courtesy of Dr Julie Cooke).

be no sign of a palpable mass. Exfoliated malignant cells in a nipple discharge appear to be associated more often with *in situ* carcinoma than with invasive malignancy.

The histological specimen usually shows ductal carcinoma *in situ* in large ducts near the nipple (Fig. 6.23). The nipple discharge specimen is usually very cellular with large clumps of carcinoma cells as well as dissociated malignant cells. The usual criteria of malignancy apply, namely increased cellularity, cell dissociation, cellular and nuclear enlargement, pleomorphism, irregularity of nuclear outline and hyperchromasia with coarse clumps of chromatin (Figs 6.24 and 6.25). 'Cupping' of cells one within another, is a feature that is sometimes seen [8]. The smears also show debris and abundant foamy macrophages (Fig. 6.26). Erythrocytes are frequently present but it must be remembered that they are also seen in the blood-stained discharges associated with benign duct papillomas.

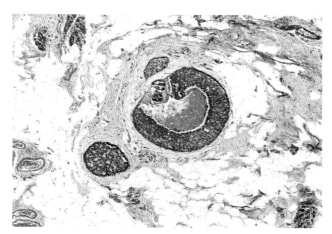

Figure 6.23 Histology of ductal carcinoma *in situ*. This section shows *in situ* carcinoma within large ducts. Note the necrotic debris in the duct lumen and the microcalcification (H & E).

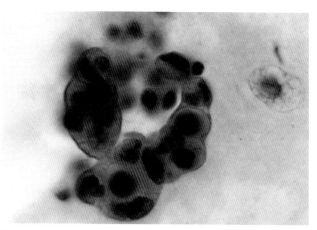

Figure 6.24 Cytology of ductal carcinoma *in situ*. This nipple discharge smear shows carcinoma cells with some foamy macrophages and erythrocytes in the background. Much care must be taken to differentiate malignant cells from the atypia commonly seen in duct papillomas (Pap). Compare with Fig. 6.19.

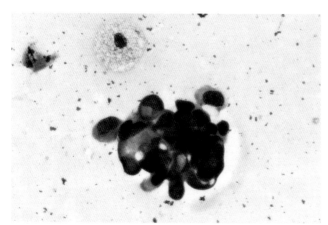

Figure 6.25 Cytology of ductal carcinoma *in situ*. This air-dried smear shows a cluster of cohesive carcinoma cells which are pleomorphic and hyperchromatic. Note the foamy macrophage in the background. These accompany both benign and malignant nipple discharge smears (MGG).

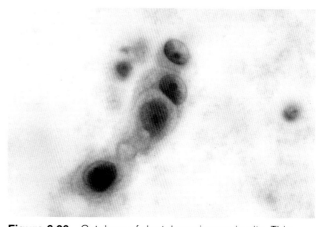

Figure 6.26 Cytology of ductal carcinoma *in situ*. This group of carcinoma cells shows 'cupping' which is a feature that may also be seen in nipple discharge specimens from duct papillomas. Note the prominent nucleoli in these malignant cells (Pap).

PAGET'S DISEASE OF THE NIPPLE

This malignant lesion is named after Sir James Paget who first described it in 1874. Clinically there is eczematous involvement of the nipple, sometimes accompanied by itching and a blood-stained discharge. Underlying ductal carcinoma is usually present. It has also been reported in conjunction with lobular, medullary and papillary carcinoma of the breast [14]. It may occur in the male breast also and can mimic melanoma [15]. Patients with Paget's disease who have palpable masses tend to have underlying invasive carcinoma and a poorer prognosis than those without palpable lesions, the latter being more likely to have *in situ* disease.

Histology shows that the epithelium of the nipple is invaded by large carcinoma cells with abundant pale cytoplasm (Fig. 6.27). They may also be seen invading the sebaceous glands as well as the terminal parts of the lactiferous ducts. There is often an associated inflammatory infiltrate.

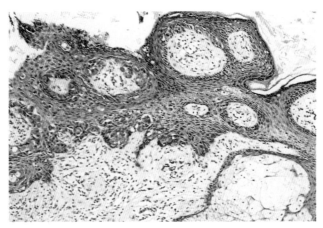

Figure 6.27 Histology of Paget's disease of the nipple. This section of nipple show squamous epithelium infiltrated by large carcinoma cells with clear cytoplasm (H & E).

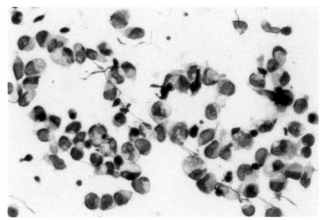

Figure 6.29 Cytology of Paget's disease. The air-dried smear shows better cell preservation. This cellular nipple scrape smear contains many single large carcinoma cells with abundant cytoplasm confirming the clinical impression of Paget's disease (MGG).

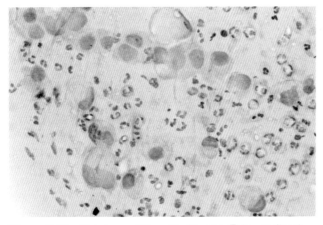

Figure 6.28 Cytology of Paget's disease. This wet-fixed nipple scrape smear shows marked air-drying artefact. This is quite common in this condition. The clusters of cells seen here show nuclear enlargement with apparently clear cytoplasm which can only be reported as 'suspicious', i.e. C4, rather than frankly malignant. Note the anucleate squames in the background (Pap).

In a detailed study of a case of Paget's disease of the nipple, Toker [16] showed that the spread of tumour cells from the ductal carcinoma to the nipple was by intraepithelial permeation of a single duct system with preservation of both the superficial layer of epithelium and the basement membrane. It has also been demonstrated that there is *in situ* transformation of epidermal cells to Paget cells [17].

A gentle scrape of the affected nipple will usually produce sufficient material for diagnostic purposes [18], but better samples are obtained after wetting the nipple with a warm saline-soaked gauze-pad for

three minutes [19]. This prevents the air drying artefact often seen in wet-fixed scrapes of the nipple [19]. The smears show many squames, debris and large carcinoma cells with abundant cytoplasm. They have hyperchromatic, irregular nuclei and may be binucleate (Figs 6.28 and 6.29).

ACKNOWLEDGEMENTS

The author gratefully thanks Dr Julie Cooke for kindly providing and describing all the mammographic pictures used, and Mrs Jennifer Walker for her uncomplaining patience in typing the several versions of the manuscript, also to the technical staff in the department who managed time after time to find slides that had been misplaced. Last but not least, the author's gratitude is extended to the Jarvis Breast Screening Unit and the Breast Surgical Team who provided most of the cytological specimens illustrated in this chapter and the one on benign appearances (Chapter 2).

REFERENCES

1. Kleinberg, D. L., Gordon, L. N., Andrew, G. and Frantz, G. (1977) Galactorrhea: A study of 2235 cases, including 48 with pituitary tumors. *New Engl. J. Med.* **296**, 589–600.
2. Fung, A., Rayter, Z., Fisher, C. *et al.* (1990) Preoperative cytology and mammography in patients with single-duct nipple discharge treated by surgery. *Br. J. Surg.* **77**, 1211–2.

3. Leif, R. C., Bobitt, D., Railey, C. *et al.* (1980) Centrifugal cytology of nipple aspirate cells. *Acta Cytol.* **24**, 255–61.

4. Sartorius, O. W., Smith, H. S., Morris, P. *et al.* (1977) Cytologic evaluation of breast fluid in the detection of breast disease. *J. Natl. Cancer Inst.* **39**, 1073–80.

5. Wrennsch, M. R., Petrakis, N. L., King, E. B. *et al.* (1992) Breast cancer incidence in women with abnormal cytology in nipple aspirates of breast fluid. *Am. J. Epidem.* **135**, 131–41.

6. Johnson, T. L. and Kini, S. R. (1991) Cytologic and clinicopathologic features of abnormal nipple secretions: 225 cases. *Diagn. Cytopathol.* **7**, 17–22.

7. Insabato, L. (1992) Nipple secretions in breast diseases. *Diagn. Cytopathol.* **2**, 200–1.

8. Papanicolaou, G. N., Holmquist, D. G., Bader, G. M. and Falk, E. A. (1958) Exfoliative cytology of the human mammary gland and its value in the diagnosis of cancer and other diseases of the breast. *Cancer*, **11**, 377–409.

9. Sara, A. S. and Gottfried, M. R. (1987) Benign papilloma of the male breast following chronic phenothiazine therapy. *Am. J. Clin. Pathol.* **87**, 649–50.

10. Rosen, P. P. and Caicco, J. A. (1986) Florid papillomatosis of the nipple. *Am. J. Surg. Pathol.* **10**, 87–101.

11. Fornage, B. D., Farouz, M. J., Pluot, M. and Bogomoletz, W. (1991) Nipple adenoma simulating carcinoma. *J. Ultrasound Med.* **10**, 55–7.

12. Handley, R. S. and Thackray, A. C. (1962) Adenoma of nipple. *Br. J. Cancer* **16**, 187–94.

13. Bhagavan, B. S., Patchefsky, A. and Koss, L. G. (1973) Florid subareolar duct papillomatosis (nipple adenoma) and mammary carcinoma: report of three cases. *Human Pathol.* **4**, 289–95.

14. Ashikari, R., Park, K., Huvos, G. and Urban, J. A. (1971) Paget's disease of the breast. *Cancer*, **26**, 680–5.

15. Stretch, J. B., Denton, K. J., Millard, P. R. and Horak, E. (1991) Paget's disease of the male breast clinically and histopathologically mimicking melanoma. *Histopathol.* **19**, 470–2.

16. Toker, C. (1961) Some observations on Paget's disease of the nipple. *Cancer*, **14**, 653–72.

17. Sagebiel, R. W. (1969) Ultrastructural observations on epidermal cells Paget's disease of the breast. *Am. J. Pathol.* **57**, 49–64.

18. Lucarotti, M. E., Dunn, J. M. and Webb, A. J. (1994) Scrape cytology in the diagnosis of Paget's disease of the breast. *Cytopathology*, **5**, 301–5.

19. Masukawa, T., Kuzma, J. F. and Straumfjord, J. V. (1973) Cytologic detection of early Paget's disease of breast with improved cellular collection method. *Acta Cytol.* **19**, 274–8.

7. Efficacy of breast needle aspiration cytodiagnosis

Peter A. Trott

STATISTICAL ANALYSIS

The published reports of breast aspiration diagnosis generally intend to indicate the accuracy of this technique with regard to diagnosing malignant and benign breast disease. However, the statistical methods of analysis vary considerably; for example, some take into account inadequate specimens and some include equivocal or suspicious diagnoses with the positive predictive value and others do not. It is therefore appropriate to list definitions of the terms used in published material to evaluate the results of breast aspiration cytodiagnosis.

Absolute sensitivity

Absolute sensitivity refers to the number of carcinomas unequivocally diagnosed, expressed as a proportion of the total number of carcinomas aspirated. In other words it is an expression of the ability to give a positive result when cancer is present.

Complete sensitivity

Complete sensitivity is the number of carcinomas diagnosed positively as well as those with equivocal appearances (i.e. excluding carcinomas definitely negative or inadequate on aspiration cytodiagnosis) expressed as a proportion of the total numbers of carcinomas aspirated. This figure has particular relevance in stereotactic aspiration cytodiagnosis when detection rather than diagnosis is more important.

Specificity

Specificity is the number of correctly identified benign lesions expressed as a proportion of the total number of benign lesions aspirated. It is the ability to give a negative finding when cancer is absent.

Positive predictive value

Clinicians are particularly interested in the positive predictive value as it indicates the degree of confidence with which they can regard a positive result. Where it is 100 per cent the clinician will know that a C5 cytodiagnosis has always meant malignancy. If it includes equivocal diagnoses then this should be made clear, but a positive predictive value of an unequivocal positive result is the number of positive results less those that are falsely positive, expressed as a proportion of the total number of true positive results. The positive predictive value of an equivocal result is the number of equivocal results less those that are falsely suspicious, expressed as a proportion of the total number of suspicious results.

Predictive value of negative reports

The predictive value of negative reports is the number of true negatives expressed as a proportion of all negative reports including those that subsequently are revealed to be malignant. Carcinomas that are diagnosed within three years of a negative needle aspirate taken from the same area of the breast are conventionally considered false negatives [1].

False negative rate

False negative rate is the number of falsely negative results expressed as a proportion of the total number of carcinomas aspirated.

Many of these categories overlap in their attempt to provide helpful statistics for comparative analysis. So far as breast aspiration cytodiagnosis is concerned, the important statistics are the absolute sensitivity, the specificity, the positive predictive value and the negative predictive value. For example, an absolute sensitivity of 0.60 means that in a group of carcinoma cases 60 per cent were given unequivocal reports and the remainder were diagnosed as either suspicious or negative. A specificity of 0.92 means that in cases without carcinoma 8 per cent were given either falsely positive or suspicious reports. A positive predictive value of 0.99 means that 1 per cent of unequivocally positive reports were incorrect and a negative predictive value of 0.70 means that 30 per cent of negative reports come from aspirates of carcinomas presently or that are diagnosed within three years subsequently.

The problem of interval cancers and how they fit into an analysis is controversial. Those falsely negative cases that subsequently, within three years, are revealed to be carcinomas may have developed tumour after the aspirate was taken, particularly if the time interval is a long one. In the context of the breast screening programme, in which patients are screened at three-yearly intervals, this could be an 'interval' cancer that has subsequently developed or it could be a case that was missed by mammography or fine needle aspiration cytodiagnosis. As the screening programme develops, more information will emerge concerning this interesting group of cancers.

ANALYSIS OF RESULTS OF REPORTED SERIES

Table 7.1 [2] shows a list of comparative reporting data of seven large series. So far as it is possible, the same data have been extracted from each paper and presented in tabular form and a similar statistical analysis has been undertaken. This is a calculation of the absolute and complete sensitivites, specificity and positive and negative predictive values. The largest series is from Franzen and Zajick [8] who reported on 3119 cases. All the carcinomas were verified histologically and the specimens were taken by cytopathologists in the cytology clinic. Their results of 0.76 and 0.78 absolute and complete sensitivities, respectively, can be compared with those of the smaller series of Brown et al. [5] in which the aspirates were performed by pathologists. Their sensitivity figures are also very high. Indeed the highest figure of complete sensitivity of 0.94 is in the Brown series and indicates, in statistical terms, the advantages of the pathologist aspirating the tumour.

Table 7.1 Comparative reporting data

		References						
		1	2	3	4	5	6*	7
Total no. of cases	a	1671	793	1002	480	1283	3119	1181
Total with carcinoma	b	1539	228	356	276	689	1099	1014
Cytology positive	c	1031	158	295	219	481	832	500
Suspicious	d	335	26	40	9	88	30	372
Negative	e	166	31	21	6	48	206	142
Total without carcinoma	f	132	565	646	204	594	2020	167
Cytology positive	g	0	0	0	0	2	1	2
Suspicious	h	27	3	10	0	53	23	19
Negative	i	46	470	636	129	338	1464	146
Inadequate rate (%)		23	13	0	42	21	12	0
Absolute sensitivity	$\dfrac{c}{b}$	0.67	0.69	0.83	0.79	0.69	0.76	0.49
Complete sensitivity	$\dfrac{c+d}{b}$	0.89	0.81	0.94	0.83	0.83	0.78	0.86
Specificity	$\dfrac{i}{f}$	0.35	0.83	0.98	0.63	0.57	0.72	0.87
Positive predictive value	$\dfrac{c}{g+c}$	1.00	1.00	1.00	1.00	0.995	0.998	0.998
Negative predictive value	$\dfrac{i}{e+j}$	0.78	0.94	0.97	0.96	0.88	0.88	0.51

1, Eisenberg et al. [3]; 2, Powles et al. [4]; 3, Brown et al. [5]; 4, Smallwood et al. [6]; 5, Barrows et al. [7]; 6, Franzen et al. [8]; 7, Ciatto et al. [9]
*Includes cases of benign cysts.

Many papers show a positive predictive value of 100 per cent and others show a value in the high 90s. This indicates the level of the diagnostic threshold which should be geared towards only providing a diagnosis of carcinoma when this is certain. The phrase 'the interpreter should feel at ease in making such a diagnosis' [1] aptly sums up the diagnostic pathologist's attitude in this regard. Giard and Hermans [10] have highlighted the difficulties in attempting to compare the reported results of breast aspiration cytodiagnosis papers. They reviewed 29 articles in which there were a total of 31 340 aspirations. As well as sensitivity and specificity they included the likelihood ratios of four different results which included definitely malignant, suspicious, benign and unsatisfactory. The analysis showed striking differences between series in the diagnostic accuracy of aspiration cytodiagnosis. For example, patients with breast cancer had a chance of obtaining a 'definitely malignant' cytological diagnosis with an accuracy ranging from 0.35 to 0.92. It was the opinion of the authors that it is virtually impossible to infer general characteristics from such an analysis because of the differences in methods and different biases. This is because the test is highly operator dependent and therefore subject to local variations.

AUDIT GUIDELINES AND QUALITY ASSURANCE

Although quality assurance is well established in gynaecological cytology it is in its infancy in breast aspiration cytodiagnosis. The establishment and development of the National Health Service Breast Screening Programme has stimulated consideration of statistical targets that should be achieved [1]. Those that are recommended in conjunction with the screening programme include an inadequate rate of less than 25 per cent, a false positive rate of less than 1 per cent and a false negative rate of less than 5 per cent. Complete sensitivity should be more than 80 per cent and specificity more than 60 per cent. Although no figure have been issued with regard to the diagnosis of surgical cases, a positive predictive value of only 95 per cent whereby 5 out of 100 categorically C5 diagnoses are incorrect, would be unacceptable particularly in those units in which primary medical therapy is used. In these cases a positive predictive value of more than 99 per cent should be attained.

So far as false positive reports are concerned, Jatoi and Trott [11] found four misdiagnoses of carcinoma in an analysis of 1104 cases of positive breast aspirates seen consecutively over a four-year period. This is an incidence of 0.36 per cent and a positive predictive value of 99.6%. The benign conditions that led to false positive diagnosis were radiation-induced changes, granulomatous mastitis and fibroadenoma.

REFERENCES

1. National Health Service Breast Screening Programme. (1993) Guidelines for cytology procedures and reporting in breast cancer screening. *NHSBSP Publication No. 23*, p. 35.
2. Trott, P. A. (1993) In *Fine Needle Aspiration Cytopathology*. (ed. J. A. Young) Blackwell, Oxford, p. 94.
3. Eisenberg, A. J. (1986) Preoperative aspiration cytology of breast tumors. *Acta Cytol.* 30, 135–46.
4. Powles, T. J., Trott, P. A. and Cherryman, G. (1991) Fine needle aspiration cytodiagnosis as a prerequisite for primary medical treatment of breast cancer. *Cytopathology*, 2, 7–12.
5. Brown, L. A., Coghill, S. B. and Powis, S. A. J. (1991) Audit of diagnostic accuracy of FNA cytology specimens taken by the histopathologist in a symptomatic breast clinic. *Cytopathology*, 2, 1–7.
6. Smallwood, J., Herbert, A. and Guyer, P. (1985) Accuracy of aspiration cytology in the diagnosis of breast disease. *Br. J. Surg.*, 72, 841–3.
7. Barrows, G. H., Anderson, T. J., Lamb, J. L. and Dixon, J. M. (1986) Fine needle aspiration of breast cancer. *Cancer*, 58, 1493–8.
8. Franzen, S. L. and Zajicek, J. (1968) Aspiration biopsy in diagnosis of palpable lesions of the breast. Critical review of 3479 consecutive biopsies. *Acta Radiol.* 7, 241–62.
9. Ciatto, S., Cecliani, S. and Grazzini, G. (1989) Positive predictive value of fine needle aspiration cytology of breast lesions. *Acta Cytol.* 33, 894–8.
10. Giard, R. W. M. and Herman, J. O. (1992) The value of aspiration cytologic examination of the breast: a statistical review of the medical literature. *Cancer*, 69, 2104–10.
11. Jatoi, G. and Trott, P. A. (1994) False-positive reporting in breast fine aspiration cytology: incidence and causes. *Breast*, in press.

8. Image-guided fine needle aspiration of impalpable breast lesions

Joan Lamb and Euphemia McGoogan

INTRODUCTION

The widespread use of mammography both as a screening test for cancer and as part of the investigation and follow-up of symptomatic breast disease, has led to the detection of increasing numbers of mammographic abnormalities. By reason of small size or lack of textural differences from the surrounding breast tissue, many of these are impalpable. This chapter aims to summarize the investigation of these lesions emphasizing aspects of particular interest to the cytopathologist.

Initially, the main burden of selecting those abnormalities most likely to be malignant, rests with the radiologist. Mammograms, produced by skilled radiographers with special training, are examined for any variation from the 'normal' or 'usual' patterns. This is a subjective assessment and requires considerable expertise. Where possible a comparison is made with any previous mammograms, a 'new' or 'changing' abnormality being regarded as potentially more significant. Additional mammography with magnification views and ultrasound examination is then used in selected patients to help to characterize any suspect areas. Benign lesions such as cysts or fibroadenomas are relatively common among impalpable abnormalities, and most are confidently identified at this stage by the radiologist, without further investigation. When assessing apparently impalpable abnormalities there is a definite place for physical examination of the breast by an experienced clinician. With the benefit of all the radiological and ultrasound information, the impalpable may become palpable, or the coexistence of palpable and impalpable lesions noted. The combined results of these procedures may be sufficient to allay suspicion of malignancy and allow reassurance of the patient, or indicate the need for further investigation.

Fine needle aspiration cytodiagnosis (FNAC) is already well established in the evaluation and management of palpable breast lesions [1, 2]. Combined with clinical and radiological findings in a triple approach, it is important in cancer diagnosis and in the selection of cases for biopsy, where it provides an opportunity for early preoperative planning of patient management and a reduced diagnostic biopsy rate. In order to extend these advantages to impalpable abnormalities, image guidance techniques have been developed to direct the aspiration needle.

In the UK the introduction of techniques to localize impalpable areas of breast tissue [3] for excision biopsy was stimulated by the needs of the UK Trial of Early Detection of Breast Cancer in the late 70s [4] rather later than in some European centres, particularly Scandinavia [5]. Following the development of improved technology the UK National Health Service Breast Screening Programme was introduced in 1988 based on the Forrest Report [6]. Many centres are still in a 'learning phase' with image guided techniques for FNAC, and it is generally accepted that their use should be monitored and only attempted in centres already experienced in the assessment of symptomatic breast disease. While it is important to detect as many cancers as early as possible to try to reduce the mortality from breast cancer [7], the number of biopsies performed for benign disease should be

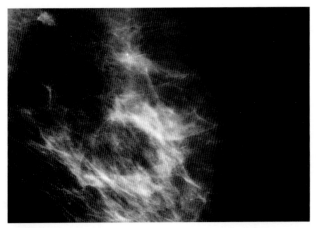

Figure 8.1 Mammogram showing a small irregular opacity.

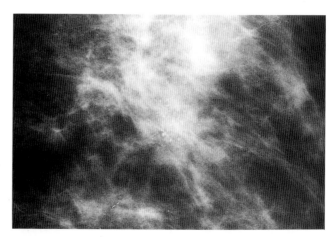

Figure 8.2 Magnified area of fine calcification seen on mammography.

low, particularly when screening asymptomatic women. A measure of quality assurance is the level of the benign:malignant biopsy ratio [8]. Levels 1:2 or 3 have been obtained in some screening centres with an occasional centre achieving 1:6 or 7 [9].

Apart from screening programmes, impalpable radiographic abnormalities are also detected during the follow-up of breast cancer patients and sometimes as a chance finding during the investigation of a palpable lesion. The radiological features of impalpable lesions are increased density (Fig. 8.1) and calcification (Fig. 8.2) or combinations of the two.

Calcification is commonly seen in mammograms and most is identified as benign by the radiologist without further investigation [10]. However, areas of small 'fine' calcifications which may be arranged in clusters or in a linear fashion, are less certainly innocent in nature so that criteria have been developed to assist in selecting those cases requiring FNAC. Calcification without opacity presents a less compact target for sampling its dispersal within an area of breast tissue, making it difficult to locate. A high inadequate or acellular rate is expected for such calcification and more needle passes may be necessary in order to assure the radiologist that the area has been thoroughly sampled. It has been noted [11] that when sufficient cells are obtained from an area of calcification, the diagnostic success equals that for opacities and combined abnormalities. It was also found that an inadequate specimen from an area carefully sampled, with each needle pass checked for cellularity, could be helpful in patient management by excluding malignancy.

METHODS OF IMAGE GUIDANCE

Two main methods of image guidance are used to direct aspiration needles and the method chosen in each case will depend on the type of mammographic abnormality. Each type may correlate with a benign or malignant lesion. The methods are ultrasound and X-ray guidance.

Ultrasound guidance

Ultrasonography has, for a long time, been helpful in obtaining information about the nature of palpable lumps [12, 13], i.e. whether they are cystic (Fig. 8.3) or solid (Figs 8.4 and 8.5), and is becoming increasingly useful in the localization of impalpable opacities. Ultrasound does not emit harmful radiation and is relatively comfortable for the patient as there is no compression of the breast. The needle is

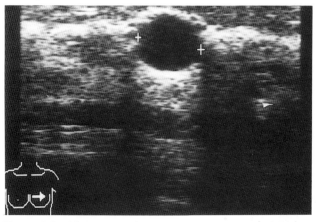

Figure 8.3 Ultrasound of a lucent oval area consistent with a benign cyst.

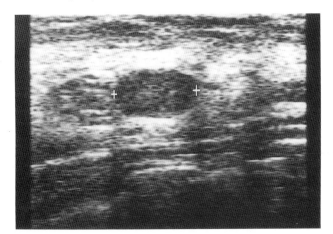

Figure 8.4 Ultrasound of an oval area with soft tissue echoes consistent with a fibroadenoma.

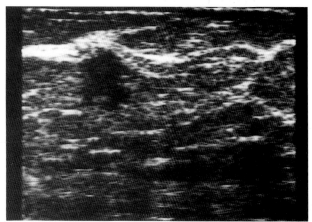

Figure 8.5 Ultrasound of a lucent area with irregular margins – suspicious of malignancy.

guided into the lesion under real-time control where it and any changes in the texture of the tissue can be seen. However, a very small, firm or mobile lesion may be difficult to needle using this method.

X-ray guidance

Of the X-ray guided procedures available, stereotaxis rather than standard methods using coordinate grids or perforated plates is recommended and is tending to replace these earlier techniques. Stereotaxis gives a third dimension to the localization of the suspect area of breast tissue and the opportunity for greater accuracy. This is supported by the report of Lofgren *et al.* [14] who found a decreased 'insufficient specimen' rate of 25 per cent using stereotaxic aspiration cytodiagnosis compared with 36 per cent using a fenestrated compression plate [15]. However, the success of any method will always depend partly on its application in the local situation and Evans and Cade [16] in a comparative trial have shown that needle placement guided by ultrasonography may be as accurate as stereotaxis.

X-ray guidance is a lengthy procedure taking on average 20–30 minutes. It is the method of choice for calcifications as these are generally regarded as being poorly visualized on ultrasound although Rizzatto [17] reported that 58 per cent of calcifications could be demonstrated sonographically. However, in the authors' experience, radiologists have found that image guidance stereotaxis is required to sample small areas of fine calcification and also small opacities or combined lesions, difficult to identify on ultrasound examination.

Of two machines used for stereotaxis, 'Mammotest' has been popular in Scandinavia and the US, but 'Stereotix' is being used more in the UK. For 'Mammotest', the woman lies prone on a trolley, her breast suspended through an opening, while for 'Stereotix', she sits at the machine with her breast pushed forward and compressed between two plastic plates. The upper plate has a rectangular window cut into it and the X-ray tube is positioned on a column which can be swung through 60°, allowing films of the same area to be taken from two angles (Figs 8.6 and 8.7). Using three dimensions a computer calculates the location of the lesion. The needle holder can then be accurately positioned and the needle tip passed directly into the lesion. Further films are taken to confirm that the patient has not moved during the procedure. Although compression helps to immobilize the lesion and facilitates sampling, the patient is required to maintain an uncom-

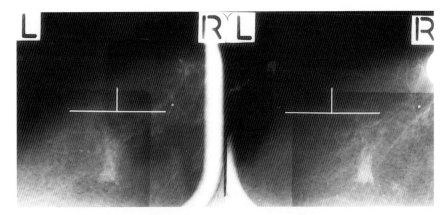

Figure 8.6 Stereotactic technique localizing a small opacity.

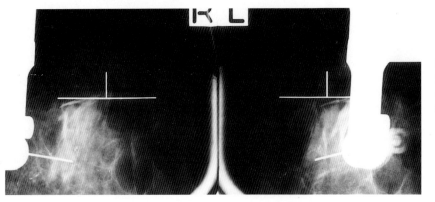

Figure 8.7 Stereotactic technique localizing an area of fine calcification, showing the cannula of the needle.

fortable position without moving. Rarely, anxiety plus the upright position used with 'Stereotix' results in fainting.

FACTORS AFFECTING DIAGNOSTIC SUCCESS IN IMPALPABLE ABNORMALITIES

Diagnostic success of impalpable breast lesions [18] has been found to depend on several factors including: (1) the skill of the radiologist; (2) preparation of aspirated material and its immediate assessment for adequacy; (3) the histology of the lesion; and (4) the combined triple 'team' approach. Similar factors operate when dealing with palpable abnormalities but are less critical.

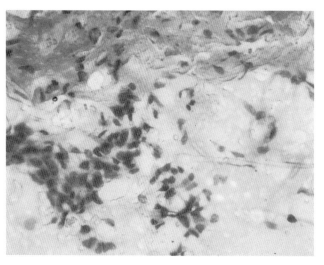

Figure 8.8 FNAC stained with Toluidine Blue showing a sheet of epithelial cells and adjacent stromal tissue.

Skill of the radiologist

The skill of the radiologist lies in selecting the abnormalities most likely to be malignant, assigning a low or high degree of suspicion to each, and sampling the area properly through the tip of the needle. The material aspirated from impalpable lesions during image guided procedures is in general much less cellular than that obtained from palpable lumps [19], and aspirates categorized as inadequate are more common. Azavedo [5] with the Scandinavian group's considerable experience, reached levels which compare well with palpable lesions.

Preparation of material and immediate assessment of adequacy of the specimen

Multiple specimens or 'passes' of the needle into the suspect area are usually required, and with relatively small aspiration samples, careful preparation becomes even more important [20]. During ultrasound-guided procedures one or two passes may be sufficient, whereas three or more are likely to be needed in cases undergoing stereotaxis.

In order to assist the radiologist in achieving a good representative sample, it is advisable to check the cellularity of each sample immediately, giving an opportunity for further passes with, if necessary, repositioning of the patient. Cells thinly smeared on a slide can be made easily recognizable using an instant stain such as Toluidine Blue (Fig. 8.8). When the cytopathologist is satisfied that sufficient material has been obtained or the radiologist decides that sampling has been as thorough as possible, the procedure can be halted. Conventional staining of the same smears follows to allow full reporting of all the material.

Both Papanicolaou and May–Grünwald Giemsa staining techniques can be used with greatly reduced time schedules to enable a final report to be available during the same clinic session. Details of preparation and staining tend to depend on personal preferences and experience, but a suggested routine would be, two smears from each pass, one stained by the Papanicolaou technique and the other by the May–Grünwald Giemsa method.

Calcified material is not often seen on smears but when present it is useful in judging the accuracy of sampling. Calcification is usually haematoxyphylic and it is therefore easily recognizable when stained by the Papanicolaou method. Occasionally calcification is composed of calcium oxalate dihydrate (Weddellite) rather than the usual calcium phosphate. Weddellite is not haematoxyphylic and was identified in 7.3 per cent of cases of mammographic calcifications in a series of breast biopsies [21].

The histology of the lesion

The cytology of a wide variety of breast lesions has already been described in previous chapters, and the criteria for the cytodiagnosis of malignancy discussed. The range of appearances, and the definitions of reporting categories are the same for palpable and impalpable lesions with the same limitations operating due to an absence of tissue architecture. Aspirates from impalpable abnormalities often provide fewer cells requiring a more critical assessment and as a result, they may be less easily designated as definitively malignant or benign and a higher proportion are likely to be reported as 'suspicious' than is found in the investigation of palpable lumps.

Furthermore, the range of histopathological diagnoses is not the same for palpable and impalpable lesions, certain histopathological lesions are found more often in impalpable lesions. Thus invasive lesions are more often well differentiated and there is a higher proportion of *in situ* cancers in mammographic lesions which tend to be smaller than palpable ones. Also, complex benign lesions, such as radial scar are comparatively common.

Table 8.1 shows the correlation of the type of mammographic abnormality with the counterpart histopathology in a group of 150 biopsies received following stereotactic FNAC in 1990/91 and Table 8.2 lists the range of detailed histopathological diagnoses found in this series.

Table 8.3 gives the diagnoses of a group of mammographic opacities sampled by ultrasound-guided FNAC from the same unit. The use of this method of guidance is increasing and in the same unit the number of such procedures more than doubled in 1992.

It can be seen in Table 8.1, that both types of mammographic abnormality yielded a high proportion of cancers, and as expected, most of the *in situ* cancers were in the 'calcification only' group. There were no *in situ* cancers detected by ultrasound-guided FNAC as shown in Table 8.3.

In the histopathological diagnoses listed in Table 8.2, there are comparatively few cysts and fibroadenomas. These appear as benign-looking rounded opacities on mammography and are relatively common among impalpable lesions. FNAC is therefore not often required for these lesions although some cysts are aspirated under ultrasound guidance.

When aspirated because of doubtful X-ray or ultrasonic features, the cytology is similar to that seen in palpable lesions. Fibroadenomas are often fibrous and poorly cellular. Some invasive cancers have well defined borders and present a rounded appearance on X-ray similar to a cyst or fibroadenoma. They will usually be infiltrating ductal carcinoma of no special type, but occasionally a medullary or mucinous carcinoma may occur. In this latter type, the smears will show 'mucoid' material in the background, not to be confused with the 'myxoid' material appearing occasionally in a fibroadenoma where there is a prominent myxoid stroma.

Other benign lesions give aspirates similar to those seen in their palpable counterparts. However with less material to assess, the presence of a few atypical or suspicious cells may make diagnosis difficult, contributing to the higher 'suspicious' rate in image-guided FNAC. On excision biopsy a few of these will be shown to be atypical ductal or lobular hyperplasia or lobular carcinoma *in situ*, adjacent to or part of an otherwise benign target lesion.

Impalpable opacities with irregular stellate outlines are recognized as highly suspicious of malignancy on mammography. They tend to be small, of the order of 10 mm or less, and are often well-differentiated cancers, in particular of the tubular type. This, and the counterpart benign lesion, radial scar or complex sclerosing lesion will be described in detail.

INVASIVE TUBULAR CANCER

These are mostly about 10 mm in diameter and at least 90 per cent of the tumour mass is composed of tubular structures lined by a single layer of small regular epithelial cells invading stroma (Fig. 8.9).

Table 8.1 Image-guided FNAC – stereotaxis. Correlation of mammographic abnormality with pathology (150 biopsies, 1990/91)

Histopathology	Mammographic abnormality		Total
	Calcification only	Opacity and calcification	
Invasive cancer	18	46	64
In situ cancer	40	8	48
Benign	24	14	38
Total	82	68	150

Table 8.2   Image-guided FNAC – stereotaxis. Histopathological diagnoses (150 biopsies, 1990/1991)

Histopathology	Total
Benign	
Fibroadenoma	3
Cyst	1
Radial scar/complex sclerosing lesion	7
Sclerosing adenosis	1
Involutional change	3
Non-proliferative hyperplasia/ fibrocystic disease	21
Atypical ductal hyperplasia	1
Atypical lobular hyperplasia	1
Total benign	38
Malignant	
Invasive cancer	
No special type	52
Tubular	6
Cribriform	1
Tubular variants	4
Lobular	1
In situ cancer	
Comedo (+solid)	29
Cribriform	4
Micropapillary	4
Mixed	10
Lobular carcinoma in situ*	1
Total malignant	112

*Incidental finding

Table 8.3   Image-guided FNAC – ultrasound (27 biopsies, 1991)

Histopathology	Total
Benign	
Fibroadenoma	2
Radial scar/complex sclerosing lesion	1
Non-proliferative hyperplasia/fibrocystic disease	6
Total benign	9
Malignant	
Invasive carcinoma	
No special type	16
Tubular	1
Tubular variant	1
In situ carcinoma	0
Total malignant	18

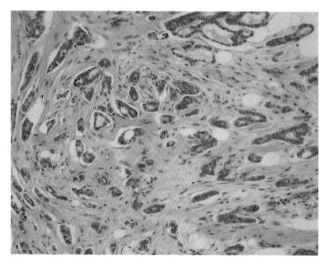

Figure 8.9 Histology of invasive cancer of tubular type.

The stroma itself is different to that usually seen associated with benign lesions being looser and showing focal elastosis.

At low power, the ctyology (Fig. 8.10) shows cohesive sheets of epithelial cells usually without regular 'bare nuclei' but with abnormally-shaped groups of tubular structures. At higher power (Fig. 8.11) only minor nuclear changes are seen and there is occasional patchy loss of cohesion.

RADIAL SCAR/COMPLEX SCLEROSING LESION

This is a benign lesion which can have a similar appearance to carcinoma on mammography, and even macroscopically on biopsy. However, the centre of the lesion is often less dense radiologically and the degree of suspicion consequently lower.

The histology shows an area of central sclerosis

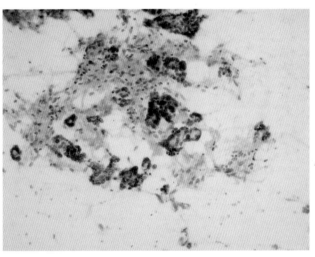

Figure 8.10 Cytology of abnormally shaped, sometimes tubular groups of epithelial cells with background stromal cells and cell fragments from a tubular cancer.

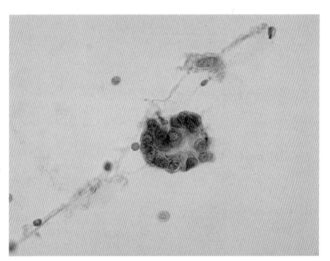

Figure 8.11 High-power view of one tubular structure.

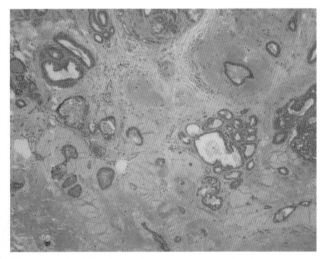

Figure 8.12 Histology of complex sclerosing lesion.

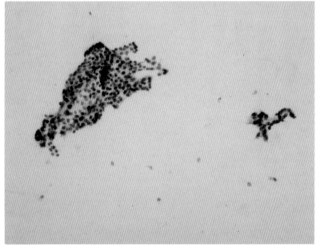

Figure 8.13 Cytology – low-power view of epithelial sheets from a complex sclerosing lesion.

with varying degrees of epithelial proliferation, apocrine metaplasia and cystic change (Fig. 8.12). The lesion is defined according to size, radial scars being arbitrarily separated from complex sclerosing lesions which are more than 10 mm in diameter. Size and age have been shown to be important with regard to the associated presence of carcinoma. In a series of 126 complex sclerosing lesions and radial scars, carcinoma of various types was seen in lesions more than 7 mm in diameter and in women aged more than 50 years [22].

At low power, the cytology (Fig. 8.13) usually shows cohesive sheets of epithelial cells with a background of bare nuclei. Apocrine and foam cells may be present. Some nuclear variation and a few abnormally shaped groups (Fig. 8.14) or tubular structures similar to those described in tubular cancers may occur.

Therefore the differential diagnosis of a small impalpable stellate opacity can be difficult on cytology, and it is not surprising that a higher proportion are put into a 'suspicious' category. Bondeson and Lindholm [23] were able to call 50 per cent of tubular cancers malignant on cytology. This compares well with a series from Edinburgh [24] in which it was noted that about a third of a mixed group of palpable and impalpable radial scar/complex sclerosing lesions were called 'suspicious' on cytology.

In situ carcinomas of ductal type are common among impalpable lesions, because they tend to produce characteristic calcification. Histological subtypes [25] have been described namely comedo, solid, micropapillary, cribriform, and mixed type.

COMEDO

This is the most common type, and the one thought most likely to become invasive.

Typically the comedo type (Fig. 8.15) has a distinctive pattern on histology of rounded, expanded ductules lined by large pleomorphic malignant cells with central necrosis and calcification. These features are mirrored in the cytology (Figs 8.16 and 8.17) and if well sampled there will be no difficulty in diagnosing malignancy on cytological grounds. The epithelial cells usually show the typical features of malignancy with enlargement, marked pleomorphism, poor cohesion and marked nuclear abnormality. These cells are often accompanied by streaks of necrotic debris and fragments of calcified material.

Although typical radiological and cytological features in keeping with *in situ* carcinoma are seen [26], invasive carcinoma is not excluded. Histological assessment is required to provide the architecture of the lesion.

OTHER TYPES

The solid type has expanded ductules filled with less pleomorphic cells than the comedo type, and without central necrosis. However it is usually part of a mixed lesion.

The micropapillary type tends to produce rather rounded groups of quite pleomorphic malignant cells and may well show some necrosis and fragments of calcified material. Often it is multifocal.

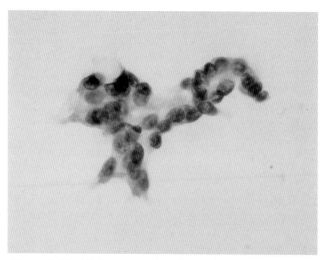

Figure 8.14 High power view of one of the groups from a complex sclerosing lesion which is abnormally shaped.

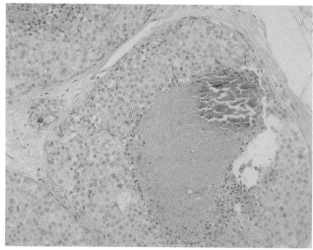

Figure 8.15 Histology of *in situ* cancer of the comedo type.

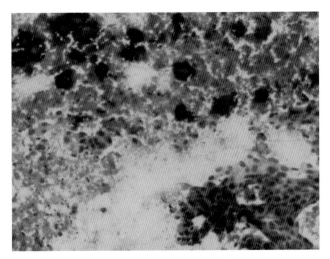

Figure 8.16 Cytology – necrosis, calcification and malignant epithelial cells from comedo *in situ* cancer.

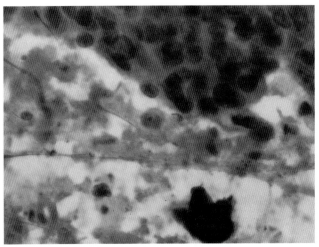

Figure 8.17 High power view of Fig. 8.16.

In contrast, *in situ* carcinoma of the cribriform type shows cohesive sheets of regular epithelial cells of usual size. Helpful features in recognizing these as malignant or suspicious of malignancy are a relative increase in the number of cells expected, without an accompanying increase in background, regular bare nuclei, and importantly, marked crowding of the cells in the sheets, plus hyperchromatism of the nuclei and some increase in granularity of the chromatin.

THE COMBINED TRIPLE 'TEAM' APPROACH

Success in the diagnosis and management of impalpable breast lesions requires strict application of the triple approach and is dependent upon clinicians, radiologists and cytopathologists working together as a 'team' [27], each being particularly aware of the strengths and weaknesses of their own discipline and able to contribute to a combined assessment. They need the assistance of skilled radiographers, cytotechnicians and nurse counsellors, and the procedure will be most successful if they can all be present together at an Assessment Clinic, discussing and sharing decisions on patient management at the time of the investigation. This approach also expedites action in each case and the patient can be informed of any plans and given choices immediately. If local factors make this difficult to achieve,

regular case discussion and real co-operation between the team members is still essential for proper patient management.

MANAGEMENT OPTIONS

The four management options are: (1) definitive planned treatment; (2) selection for diagnostic biopsy; (3) early recall for reassessment; and (4) reassurance and discharge from the clinic. In the case of a patient screened under the NHS Breast Screening Programme (currently between the ages of 50 and 64 years) she will return to routine three-yearly screening.

An option is chosen by the team after weighing up the available information which will include patient history, clinical examination, the degree of suspicion on X-ray and ultrasound, the possibility of multifocality, confidence in the achievement of a representative sample for FNAC and the cytopathology result.

A high degree of suspicion on radiology usually overrides a cytopathology result in the benign or inadequate categories and supports advocating diagnostic biopsy, whereas a low degree of suspicion on radiology may be even further reduced by a 'benign' or 'inadequate' result, allowing early recall or complete reassurance for the patient. Some workers regard the 'inadequate' category as 'no result'. However when it follows careful sampling by a radiolgist confident of the needle placement and supported by immediate cellularity checking of the aspirate, it is useful in patient management.

If a diagnosis of malignancy is made on combined assessment of a small impalpable lesion, treatment can be planned and if the presence of a benign lesion is confirmed the patient can be discharged from the clinic or returned to routine screening. The sensitivity of the procedure needs more time for assessment and must take into account the appearance of interval cancers.

In the context of the National Health Service Breast Screening Programme interval cancers are those presenting during the three years between mammographic screening intervals [28]. These are a mixed group, of which more than half have turned out to be new cancers (i.e. not visible on review of the previous mammorgram), approximately one quarter are 'missed' cancers (i.e. not seen on the previous mammogram because of technical or observer error), the remainder being radiographically permanently occult.

ACKNOWLEDGEMENT

Reproductions of mammograms are by courtesy of Dr B. Muir.

REFERENCES

1. Zajdela, A., Chossein, N. A. and Pilleston, J. P. (1975) The value of aspiration cytology in the diagnosis of breast cancer. *Cancer*, **35**, 499–506.
2. Dixon, J. M., Anderson, T. J., Lamb, J. *et al.* (1984) Fine needle aspiration cytology in relationship to clinical examination and mammography in the diagnosis of a solid breast mass. *Br. J. Surg.*, **71**, 593–6.
3. Chetty, U., Kirkpatrick, A. E., Anderson, T. J. *et al.* (1983) Localisation and excision of occult breast lesions. *Br. J. Surg.* **70**, 607–10.
4. UK Trial of Early Detection of Breast Cancer Group. (1981) Trial of early detection of breast cancer: description of method. *Br. J. Cancer*, **44**, 618–27.
5. Azavedo, E., Svane, G. and Auer, G. (1989) Stereotactic fine needle biopsy in 2594 mammographically detected non-palpable lesions. *Lancet*, **1** (8646), 1033–6.
6. Working Group (Chairman A. P. M. Forrest), Breast Cancer Screening (1987) *Women's Health Care. Report to the Health Ministers of England, Wales, Scotland and Northern Ireland*, HM Stationery Office, London, ISBN 011321071X.
7. Tabar, L., Gad, A., Holmberg, L. H. *et al.* (1985) Reduction in mortality from breast cancer after mass screening with mammography. *Lancet*, **i**, 829–32.
8. The Royal College of Radiologists (1990) *Quality Assurance Guidelines for Radiologists*. NHSBSP Screening Publications, ISBN 1 872263 208.
9. Wells, C. A., Ellis, I. O., Zakhour, H. D. and Wilson, A. R. (1994) Guidelines for cytology procedures and reporting on fine needle aspirates of the breast. Cytology subgroup of the National Co-ordinating Committee for Breast Cancer Screening Pathology. *Cytopathology*, **5**, 316–34.
10. Fajardo, L. L., Davis, J. R., Wiens, J. L. and Trego, D. C. (1990) Mammography-guided stereotactic fine needle aspiration cytology of non-palpable breast lesions; prospective comparison with surgical biopsy results. *Am. J. Roentgenol.* **155**, 977–81.
11. Muir, B., Anderson, T. J., Lamb, J. *et al.* (1992) Clustered microcalcifications in the breast: a prospective study. *Breast*, **1**, 187–92.
12. Jackson, V. P. (1990) The role of ultrasound in breast imaging. *Radiology*, **177**, 305–11.
13. Bassett, L. W. and Kumine Smith, C. (1991) Breast sonography. *Am. J. Roentgenol.* **156**, 455–69.
14. Lofgren, M., Andersson, I. and Lindholm, K. (1990) Stereotactic fine needle aspiration for cytologic diagnoses of non-palpable breast lesions. *Am. J. Roentgenol.* **154**, 1191–5.
15. Lofgren, M., Andersson, I., Bondeson, L. and Lindholm, K. (1988) X-ray guided fine needle aspiration for the cytologic diagnoses of non-palpable breast lesions. *Cancer*, **61**, 1032–7.
16. Evans, W. P. and Cade, S. H. (1989) Needle localisation and fine needle aspiration biopsy of non-palpable breast lesions with use of standard and stereotactic equipment. *Radiology*, **175**, 53–6.
17. Rizzatto, G. (1992) *Breast Cytology in Clinical Practice* (Eds S. Catania and S. Ciatto), Martin Dunitz, London, p. 95.
18. Lamb, J., Anderson, T. J., Dixon, M. J. and Levack, P. (1987) Role of fine needle aspiration cytology in breast screening. *J. Clin. Pathol.* **40**, 705–9.
19. Ciatto, S., Rosselli Del Turco, N. and Bravetti, P. (1989) Non-palpable breast lesions: stereotaxic fine-needle aspiration cytology. *Radiology*, **40**, 380–2.
20. Dent, D. N., Kirkpatrick, A. E., McGoogan, E. *et al.* (1989) Stereotaxic localisation and aspiration cytology of impalpable breast lesions. *Clin. Radiol.* **40**, 380–2.
21. Going, J. J., Anderson, T. J., Crocker, P. R. and Levison, D. A. (1990) Weddlellite calcification in the breast: eighteen cases with implications for breast screening. *Histopathology*, **16**, 119–24.
22. Sloane, J. P. and Mayers, M. M. (1993) Carcinoma and atypical hyperplasia in radial scars and complex sclerosing lesions: importance of lesion size and patient age. *Histopathology*, **23**, 225–31.
23. Bondeson, L. and Lindholm, K. (1990) Aspiration cytology of tubular breast carcinoma. *Acta Cytol.* **34**, 15–20.
24. Lamb, J. and McGoogan, E. (1994) Fine needle aspiration cytology of breast of tubular type and in radial scar/complex sclerosing lesions. *Cytopathology*, **5**, 17–26.

25. Bellamy, C., McDonald, C., Salter, D. M. *et al.* (1993) Non-invasive ductal carcinoma of the breast: the relevance of histologic categorization. *Hum. Pathol.* **24** (1), 16–23.

26. Jackson, V. P. and Bassett, L. W. (1990) Stereotactic fine needle aspiration biopsy for non-palpable breast lesions. Commentary. *Am. J. Roentgenol.* **154**, 1196–7.

27. Warren, R. (1991) Team learning and breast cancer screening. *Lancet*, 338–514.

28. Peeters, P. H. M., Verbeek, A. L. M., Hendriks, J. H. C. L. *et al.* (1989) The occurrence of interval cancers in the Nijmegen Screening Programme. *Br. J. Cancer*, **59**, 929–32.

9. Research techniques and applications

Ian O. Ellis

INTRODUCTION

In the last few years pathology laboratories have seen the rapid development of novel technology including immunocytochemistry with polyclonal and monoclonal antibody production, molecular biology through nucleic acid probe methods and biomedical engineering development resulting in advanced flow and image cytometric systems. Cytopathologists have the advantage of working with a medium suitable for study by all of these techniques, many of which have potential clinical applications in disease diagnosis, classification and treatment.

In this chapter these techniques are described and illustrated using examples of ongoing research and their current or potential clinical roles.

LIGHT MICROSCOPY

Despite innovations which have occurred in recent years, the light microscope remains the standard piece of diagnostic equipment in all cytopathology laboratories. The principle role of breast needle aspiration is to establish a diagnosis of breast cancer by microscopic examination of the sample. The energies of cytopathologists have been directed towards this goal and in the past they have seldom been encouraged to extend their assessment towards further classification of disease. Features visible using routine preparations such as air-dried Giemsa stained or wet-fixed Papanicolaou stained direct smears are potentially associated with the degree of differentiation or behaviour of a tumour. In breast

Table 9.1 Details of features used in a variety of breast cancer cytological grading systems

Features considered	Mouriquand [3]	Thomas [4]	Cornelisse [5]	Kuenen-Boumeester [6]	Zajdela [7]	Mossler [8]	Wallgren [9]	Hunt [10]	Robinson [11]
Single cells with cytoplasm	–	–	–		–	–	–	–	–
Cell pattern dispersed or clumps	+	+	–	–	–	–	+	+	+
Naked nuclei	+	–	–	–	–	–	+	–	–
Nuclear pleomorphism (anisokaryosis)	+	+	–		–	–	–	+	+
Nuclear size	+	–	–	–			+	+ Compared to red blood cells	+ Compared to red blood cells
Nuclear diameter	–	Ocular micrometre	–	–	Ocular micrometre	Ocular micrometre			
Nuclear area	–	–	Image analysis morphometry	Image analysis morphometry	–	Mean calculated from above	–	–	–
Nuclear area variability	–	–	+	+		–	–	–	+
Hypo/hyperchromasia	+	–	–	–		–	–	–	+
Presence of nucleoli and their staining pattern	–	+	–				+	+	+
Mitoses	+	–	–	–	–	–	+	–	–
Stain used	Hypochromic Papanicolaou	Air-dried Dif Quick	Not stated	Air-dried MGG	Air-dried MGG	Alcohol-fixed Pap	Air-fixed Pap	Air-dried MGG	Alcohol-fixed Pap
Type of cases	Aspirates of carcinoma	Aspirates of benign and malignant cases	Imprint preparations of benign and malignant cases	Aspirates of carcinoma	Aspirates of carcinoma	Aspirates of carcinoma	Aspirates of carcinoma	Aspirates of carcinoma	Aspirates of carcinoma
Cytological grade audit	Unfavourable incidents Histological grade TNM stage	Histological diagnosis and grade Lymph node status	Histological diagnosis Age Lymph node status	Survival Distant metastases Lymph node status	TNM stage 5-year survival Disease-free interval	Oestrogen receptors	Stage Survival Histological grade	Histological grade	Histological grade
Necrosis	–	–	–	–	–	–	+	–	–

MGG = May–Grünwald Giemsa.

cancer, the morphological characteristics of the tumour seen in histological sections are generally interpreted in the form of a histological type and a histological grade. The definitions of many of the well-recognized special types of breast cancer [1, 2] rests on tissue architectural features and on the purity of the tumour. Cytology preparations have the disadvantage of reflecting many of the features of individual histological types but without the reassurance of absolute purity or indeed information about the architectural characteristics which can be seen in histological sections. Although the features associated with various types can be recognized in FNA samples, for example, lakes of mucin containing clusters of tumour cells is a feature of mucinous carcinoma, most authorities only accept 90 per cent or absolute histological purity of a special type pattern to establish this diagnosis and its favourable prognosis. A cytologist can only indicate that mucinous features are present and is unable to exclude coexistence of non-special type elements which would negate a good prognosis. Grading systems perhaps have greater potential for direct cytological/histological correlation.

Cytology grading of breast cancer

A variety of grading systems using standard cytology preparations have been described (Table 9.1). These systems have potential application in disease classification prior to treatment. Some specialist breast cancer centres are currently evaluating the use of primary (neoadjuvant) chemotherapy as a routine alternative to surgery for the treatment of primary breast cancer. This approach of using chemotherapy before any type of surgery may have long-term prognostic benefits and can reduce the size of the primary tumour to a level where conservation therapy is more feasible, thus increasing the availability of this type of surgical treatment. Identification using FNA samples of cases likely to respond to chemotherapy would be of great benefit in selecting cases for this type of treatment. Grading systems could offer this ability. The advantage of a simple but effective microscopical cytological grading system would be its economy and ease of application to routine samples.

It is current practice in Nottingham to use a simple cytological grading system (Table 9.2) relying on three cytological features which can be easily assessed in routinely prepared air-dried May–Grünwald Giemsa stained smears [10]. This system is semi-quantitative and has been validated by comparison with histological grade using Elston and Ellis's method [12]. Each cytological variable is given a numerical score, the sum of the total scores is used to determine the overall grade, either high or low (Fig. 9.1). This cytological grading system is effective in the identification of high histological grade tumours but has poor discrimination between histological grades I and II. Such a grading system could be used to identify high-grade tumours suitable for chemotherapy prior to surgery.

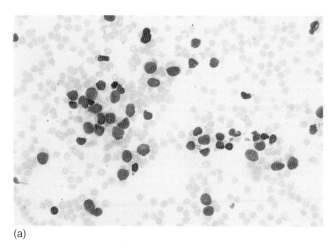

(a)

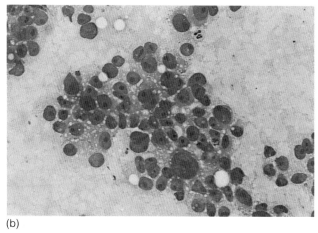

(b)

Figure 9.1 Two examples of breast cancer illustrating low grade (a) and high grade (b) cytological features photographed at the same magnification. The cells in (a) are small and show little variation in size and have small indistinct nucleoli in contrast to those in (b) which are pleomorphic with occasional very large cells (>4 red blood cells diameter) and have easily visible nucleoli.

Table 9.2   The Nottingham Breast Cytology Grading System

Nuclear diameter	
Most nuclei less than or equal to the diameter of 2 rbcs*	1
Nuclei greater than 2 rbcs but less than 4 rbcs	2
Some nuclei greater than 4 rbcs	3
Nuclear pleomorphism	
Mild	1
Moderate	2
Severe	3
Multiple, easily seen nucleoli	
Absent	0
Present	1
Low grade tumours score less than or equal to 4	
High grade tumours score greater than or equal to 5	

*rbcs = red blood cells

MORPHOMETRY AND CYTOMETRY

Microscopists routinely use subjective evaluation of morphological characteristics to enable classification or characterization of a disease process. Objective measurement of the size, shape, arrangement and tinctorial characteristics of breast tumour cell populations can provide reproducible systems for the classification of such cell populations. A variety of techniques, including standard morphometric methods, computer-assisted morphometry technology, image cytometry and flow cytometry [13–15] can be used to measure cell size and shape, nuclear size and shape, cellularity, mitotic frequency and nuclear chromatin texture and nucleolar morphology [13, 16]. Staining of nuclear DNA with stoichiometric visible or fluorescent stains allows quantitation of nuclear DNA content by flow cytometry or image cytometry. Such assessment of DNA content can be used to identify abnormalities of ploidy and to estimate the growth fraction of a cell population [17–19].

IMAGE CYTOMETRY

A variety of interactive image cytometric systems is now available commercially with appropriate software for medical laboratory use. The applications available include cell measurement, quantitation of DNA and quantitation of immunocytochemical preparations. Some systems allow the user to adapt or write software appropriate for their individual needs.

The original and the more basic current systems rely on the operator to identify appropriate cells for study and indicate the boundaries of these objects by drawing round each cell manually. Improved image systems using thresholding techniques are now commonplace and provide fully automated or semiautomated capture methods of cells, the characteristics of which can be predetermined allowing exclusion of artefacts or inappropriate cells. With ideal preparations and automated slide carrying and microscope stage systems, fully automated scanning of multiple cases is feasible. Images of individual cells of interest can be stored and displayed to an operator on request. Alternatively, an overview analysis of the entire cell population can be provided in histogram or numerical formats.

These systems have three principal groups of components (Fig. 9.2a and b):

1. image capture – usually a modified optical light microscope with attached black and white or colour solid-state camera, VDU display and enhanced PC computer (Fig. 9.2a);
2. image analysis – the PC computer with appropriate software (Fig. 9.2a); and
3. data display and analysis – VDU displays, PC computer and appropriate software (Figs 9.2b and c).

Quantitation of DNA

Quantitation of DNA using an image cytometry system relies on staining of the cell preparation with a stoichiometric DNA stain, usually of Feulgen type (Fig. 9.3). The methodology uses hydrochloric acid hydrolysis of the DNA to give sugar aldehyde residues. A dye such as thionin is coupled via the Schiff's reaction to the sugar aldehyde residues to give a colour (blue if thionin is used) (Fig. 9.3). The amount of dye coupled is directly proportional to the amount of DNA present. Quantitation of DNA is based on measuring the optical density of each image sub-unit or pixel then giving a summed optical density of all the pixels present for each cell

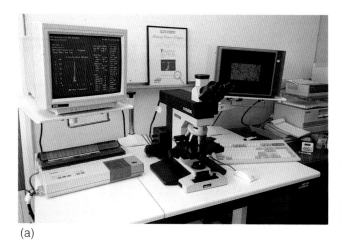

(a)

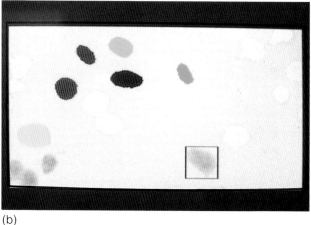

(b)

Figure 9.2 An example of an image analysis system the CAS 200 (a). The image being assessed is displayed on a VDU screen. Cells with particular characteristics can be identified through prior programming of ranges of their known characteristics (b). The data derived from the sample is displayed on a second VDU (c).

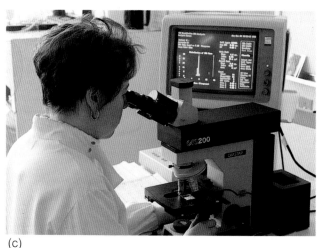

(c)

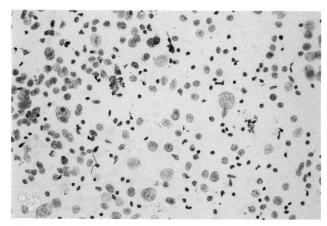

Figure 9.3 A cytospin preparation of a breast cancer needle aspirate stained with a thionin Feulgen stain for image analysis assessment of DNA and cell morphological characteristics.

nucleus in the image. Measurement of DNA in this manner is used to determine the ploidy of a population of tumour cells. Normal resting cells have the same amounts of DNA known as 2c (Fig. 9.4a). The DNA content of normal cells doubles during the cell cycle (see Fig. 9.4b) prior to cell division; hence normal cell populations have a standard biphasic DNA profile (Fig. 9.8). A population of cells with an abnormal (non 2c or 4c) DNA content (Fig. 9.4b) has major genetic/chromosomal abnormalities which are seen almost exclusively in malignant tumours. Such information can be used to contribute to a diagnosis of malignancy [20, 21] by identification of a clone of cells with a bizarre DNA content and as a system of classification and prognosis [18] (Fig. 9.5).

Cell measurement

Most image cytometry systems have cell measurement programmes which can provide rapid and objective evaluation of a wide range of cell characteristics such as cytoplasm and nucleolar size, shape, staining characteristics and texture (Fig. 9.3). These can be combined with DNA assessment to provide an image cytometric diagnostic classification system or grading system [21–24]. Such image cytometry

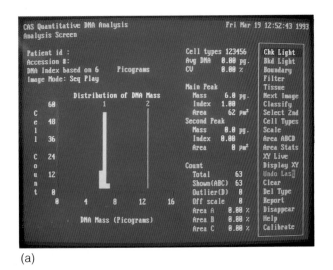

(a)

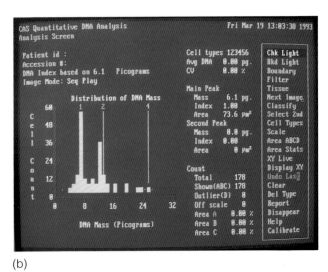

(b)

Figure 9.4 Two DNA profiles from a benign lesion (a) which has a normal 2c profile and a carcinoma (b) which has an abnormal DNA index value.

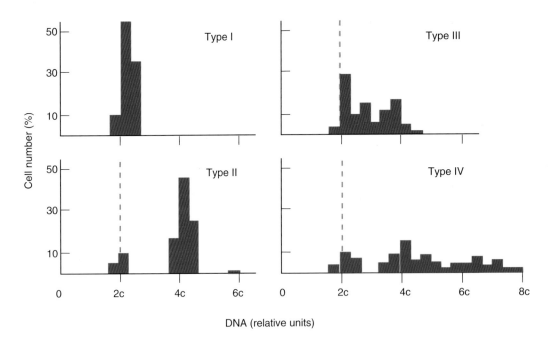

Figure 9.5 The Auer classification system of DNA histogram types. Type I: a single distinct model diploid DNA (2c) DNA peak; Type II: a single tetraploid (4c) DNA peak or two peaks at 2c and 4c; Type III: two peaks at 2c and 4c but with over 5% of cells between the peaks, i.e. a high S-phase cell population; and Type IV: distinct aneuploidy with scattered DNA value exceeding the normal 4c region.

Figure 9.6 A breast cancer FNA sample labelled by immunocytochemical staining of cytoplasmic cytokeratin (red) and Fuelgen staining of nuclear DNA (blue). An image or cytometric system can be programmed to measure nuclear DNA content of only cells with cytokeratin reactivity.

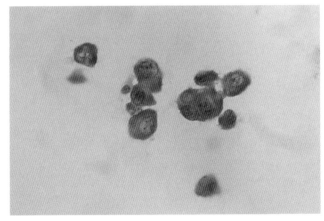

grading systems have similar potential uses to the microscopical grading systems described earlier but have the additional benefits of objectivity and potential for automation.

Immunocytochemistry quantitation

Semiautomated and automated image cytometry and flow cytometry systems can be programmed to assess a number of labelled cells or the degree of labelling in individual cells within a population of labelled cells (Fig. 9.6). This has potential benefits over standard microscopical classification being rapid and giving an objective score. For example, in breast cancer this technology has been applied to image cytometric measurement of oestrogen and progesterone receptor assessment and proliferation marker assessment [25] (see later sections on 'oestrogen receptor' and 'growth factor proliferation index').

FLOW CYTOMETRY

Flow cytometry measures the features of a cell population by passing a monodispersed sample of cells suspended in a narrow stream of fluid, between stationary detectors (Fig. 9.7). A stream of individual cells is produced by passing the sample through a fine nozzle under pressure. The end cell is surrounded and aligned by a sheath of fluid and is passed through a laser beam. The size of the individual cell can be estimated by measuring the amount of light scattered in a forward direction. Other characteristics can be assessed by prior labelling of the cells with fluorescent stains or fluorescent labelled antibodies. The laser will excite fluorescence in the stained cells, the intensity of which can be measured. In some systems a cell sorting facility is available whereby the individual cells are charged, positively or negatively, according to their characteristics and deflected according to their charge into collecting wells.

The speed of flow cytometry systems allows the measurement of thousands of cells (usually 10 000–20 000) in a matter of minutes. The resolution of individual cell measurements is poor but the ability to measure large cell populations can provide an accurate overview of the characteristics of a cell population and is particularly useful for identifying sub-populations of cells with abnormal DNA content and the distribution of cells through the cell cycle. Comprehensive reviews of the applications of flow cytometry with particular reference to DNA assessment are available [26, 27].

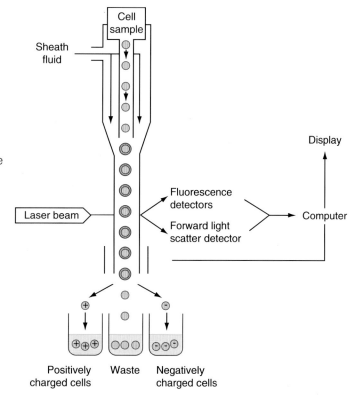

Figure 9.7 A schematic diagram of a flow cytometer with a cell-sorting facility (see text for details).

DNA analysis

The role of DNA analysis in breast disease remains controversial and was discussed briefly earlier with respect to diagnosis and classification. Flow cytometric analysis of DNA has been proposed as a system for prognostic classification of breast cancer allowing evaluation of a large number of tumour cells, thus providing a comprehensive overview of the DNA content of the tumour [18]. The cost of the equipment required for flow cytometry and the yields of cells required to provide a standard histogram have inhibited its acceptance as a routine system for the classification of breast cytology samples. It does, however, remain a powerful tool for research investigations particularly for the assessment of tumour growth fraction.

Cell cycle growth fraction measurement

Proliferating cells pass through a cyclical series of discrete phases during growth – the growth cycle (see Fig. 9.8). On completing cell division, cells can exit the cycle into a resting state G0 (gap 0) or re-enter the cycle at G1 (gap 1). These latter cells progress to the S (synthesis) phase when new DNA is produced to duplicate the chromosome numbers and then enter the second gap phase (G2). After G2, mitosis (M phase) occurs when the cell divides into two daughters each with an equal complement of chromosomes. The length of time spent in S, G2 and M is relatively constant for a particular cell type but variation may occur in the time spent in the G1 phase.

The proportion of tumour cells in the growth cycle (G1, S, G2, M) rather than in the resting state (G0) can give an indication of the potential growth of the tumour and is related to prognosis and response to chemotherapy [28]. Tumours with a high growth fraction have a poor prognosis but are more likely to show a benefit from chemotherapy. It should be borne in mind that tumour growth or doubling time is also influenced by a number of other variables including the time in growth cycle and rate of cell death [17]. Growth fraction index, unless coupled to these other measurements, cannot be used to give an accurate measurement of potential doubling time.

The most accurate system for measuring tumour growth is to allow *in vitro* uptake of a radiolabelled precursor of DNA such as thymidine or 5-bromodeoxyuridine (BRDU) an analogue of thymidine which will be incorporated into the DNA of the cells in the S-phase of the cycle [29, 30]. Labelled cells can be identified using autoradiography if radiolabelled thymidine is used or by immunocytochemistry or flow cytometry by using an anti-BRDU antibody if BRDU is used as the label [30, 31]. A single sample of tumour taken at resection can provide an S-phase fraction index but sequential sampling of tumour allows more accurate measurement of profileration through calculation of the numbers of cells entering S-phase during a given time period. Alternative less complex methods for growth fraction estimation are flow cytometric measurement of S-phase and immunocytochemical labelling using antibodies specific for cell cycle associated molecules.

The distribution of cells within the components of the cell cycle (Fig. 9.8) can be seen and measured

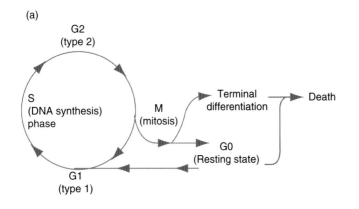
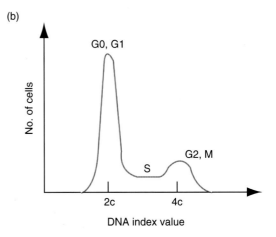

Figure 9.8 The cell cycle and related DNA histogram profile.

using flow cytometric analysis of DNA. Owing to the large number of cells measured in a flow cytometric assay, accurate identification of small cohorts of cells is possible. In particular, the proportion of cells in S-phase of the cell cycle which have a DNA content between diploid (G0 and G1) and tetraploid (G2 and M) can be identified accurately. Measurements of this type are relatively simple when the tumour cell population is diploid or has a single common DNA mass and can be used to give an indication of the growth fraction of the tumour which is related to prognosis and response to treatment. A proportion (up to 20 per cent) of breast cancers are polyploid, which means that the tumour cell population contains two or more clones of cells each of which has a different chromosome and hence DNA content. Such tumours will have multiple overlapping DNA histogram profiles which are difficult to assess except by complex mathematic modelling. Although flow cytometric measurement of S-phase fraction of a tumour cell population is a relatively accurate measurement of the growth fraction of a tumour, the problem of analysis in polyploid tumours means that a significant proportion of tumours cannot be adequately assessed.

IMMUNOCYTOCHEMISTRY

Of the various technologies described in this chapter, immunocytochemistry has had perhaps the greatest impact on investigative research of breast cancer through the development and application of monoclonal and polyclonal antibodies. Such methods have advanced the understanding of a variety of fundamental processes involving carcinogenesis and tumour cell behaviour. The majority of immunocytochemical investigations in breast cancer have been directed towards histological samples but are equally applicable to cytology samples. The types of molecules which have stimulated the most interest are shown in Table 9.3.

The techniques used for immunocytochemistry are now well established in most laboratories. Critical appraisal of immunocytochemistry techniques is beyond the scope of this chapter and the reader should refer to one of the standard textbooks [32]. Both direct smear and cytospin preparations are robust, and flexible cell preparative methods which allow adaptation of immunocytochemical techniques and fixation appropriate for the antigen are being sought. Experimentation with collection media, slide

Table 9.3   Antibodies to the following molecules have stimulated the most interest in breast cancer research

Class of molecule	Specific antibodies
Epithelial mucins	Polymorphic epithelial mucin [47, 48, 49, 50]
Growth factors and receptors	Epidermal growth factor receptor [51, 52] Transforming growth factors α and β [53, 54]
Oncogene products	c-*erb*B-2 [55, 56, 57, 58, 59] *ras* [60, 61, 62] *myc* [63]
Cell cycle markers	Thymidine (autoradiography) [28, 64] Bromodeoxyuridine [30, 31] Ki 67 [39] Proliferating cell nuclear antigen [41]
Hormone receptors	Oestrogen and progesterone receptor
Enzymes	Cathepsin-D [65, 66] Plasminogen activator [67]
Multidrug resistance gene	P-glycoprotein [43, 44]

preparation, fixation and staining method are all required when establishing a new research investigation requiring immunocytochemistry.

Oestrogen receptor

Traditionally oestrogen receptor has been assayed in breast cancer on cytosol fractions of tumour tissue homogenates using a ligand binding assay. This method has been superseded following the development of oestrogen receptor specific monoclonal antibodies [33]. These can be used in high sensitivity Enzyme Linked Immunosorbent Assays (ELISA) of tissue homogenates or in immunocytochemical assays of tissue sections or needle aspirate samples (Figs 9.9 and 9.10) [34, 35]. Although less sensitive, immunocytochemical assay has the major benefit of allowing synchronous confirmation of the presence of tumour with qualitative and semiquantitative

assessment of receptor reactivity. In addition, samples obtained by needle aspiration are generally too small for biochemical ELISA but can be routinely assessed using immunocytochemistry. Immunoreactivity can be assessed in a semiquantitative fashion using either the proportion of tumour cells stained, where cases showing over 15 per cent positive cells are regarded as oestrogen receptor positive, or the semiquantitative H-score system described in the next paragraph. Both show good correlation with biochemical assays [36].

In the H-score system the microscopist assesses in a semiquantitative fashion the proportion of positive and negative tumour cells. The positive tumour cells are then sub-categorized into those showing weak reactivity (grade I), moderate reactivity (grade II) and strong reactivity (grade III). The percentage of tumour cells showing each of these levels of reactivity is scored. To give an overall score (with a range between 0 and 300) the percentage of tumour cells in

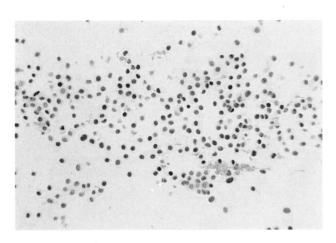

Figure 9.9 Immunocytochemical staining of oestrogen receptor in a breast fine needle aspirate sample. A streptavidin biotin method has been used with diaminobenzidine as the chromogen substrate giving a brown reaction. A green counterstain has been used to allow image analysis measurement. See Fig. 9.10.

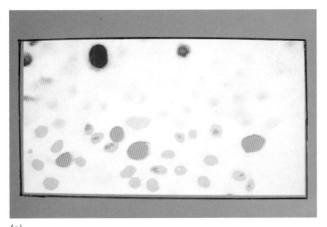

(a)

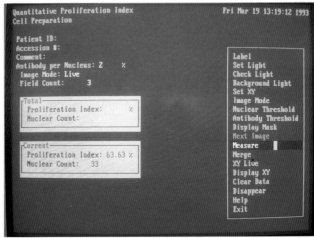

(b)

Figure 9.10 Semiautomated quantitation of an immunocytochemical oestrogen receptor assay. The

proportion of cells staining and intensity of reactivity (a) is measured by the system and the results displayed (b).

each category is multiplied by the numerical value of the grade (1, 2 or 3).

$$H\text{-score} = (\%\ \text{grade I cells} \times 1)$$
$$+ (\%\ \text{grade II cells} \times 2)$$
$$+ (\%\ \text{grade III cells} \times 3)$$

The cut-off for oestrogen receptor negative tumour cells may vary according to the clinical decision to be made but it is generally between an H-score of 50 and 100 [34, 35]. Assessment of oestrogen receptor immunoreactivity in tissue sections and cytology samples can also be assessed using an image analysis system such as the CAS 100 or 200 [25] as previously described. This system has the advantage of giving a more objective score.

Some clinical groups now use oestrogen receptor assay of fine needle aspiration samples to direct clinical decision making and help improve patient choice [35, 37]. A high proportion of elderly women presenting with primary breast cancer can respond satisfactorily to primary hormone therapy and could avoid the need for any surgery. Patients suitable for this type of medical treatment can be identified by positive receptor immunoreactivity of fine needle aspirate samples of their tumour taken at their first clinic visit. Similarly, patients presenting with advanced breast cancer require critical choice of the first form of therapy as their life expectancy is short. Some of these patients may respond to hormone therapy and such likely responders can also be identified by receptor assay of needle aspiration samples taken at their first out-patient clinic visit.

Growth fraction/proliferation index

Histological breast cancer grading systems use mitotic figure counts per unit area of section or high-power field to give an estimate of tumour growth potential. Mitotic figures are relatively infrequent (<1–10 per thousand tumour cells) and are difficult to identify accurately in cytology preparations or are disrupted during the aspiration process. These problems preclude routine counting of mitotic figures in cytology samples as an accurate method of assessing growth fraction.

Immunocytochemical staining of cytology samples with the antibodies specific for the molecules associated with cell division provides a relatively simple alternative technique for assessing growth fraction. Such antibodies include Ki 67 and MIB1 [38–40] which detect similar growth-phase-associated antigen and antibodies to proliferating cell nuclear antigen (PCNA) (also known as cyclin) [41]. PCNA is a component of the DNA polymerase-D enzyme which appears in the nucleus in late S-phase. For example a Ki 67 antibody immunocytochemistry labelling index based on a simple microscopical count (or measurement by image or flow cytometry) is associated with the growth fraction of tumour as assessed by flow cytometric measurement of S-phase fraction, histological grade and patient prognosis [38].

The use of such methods on cytology samples [42] has exciting potential for allowing early preoperative evaluation of tumours which could direct the use of neoadjuvant or primary forms of medical therapy including chemotherapy or hormone therapy, and potentially avoid or facilitate the use of surgery as the current principal method of treatment for primary breast cancer.

P-glycoprotein/multidrug resistant gene product

The use of chemotherapeutic agents is often encumbered by inherent or acquired tumour resistance to a single drug or combination of drugs. The multidrug resistant phenotype has recently been recognized to be associated with expression of a 170 kD membrane glycoprotein (p-glycoprotein) which acts as an energy-dependent pump removing certain families of chemotherapeutic drug [43]. Antibodies to p-glycoprotein have been produced which can be used to identify expression in tumour samples. Few studies have been performed in human breast cancer but the development of the multidrug resistant phenotype appears to be a late phenomenon [44].

MOLECULAR BIOLOGY

Recombinant DNA techniques of filter hybridization (blotting) and *in situ* hybridization are powerful techniques which are being used to increase the understanding of gene regulation and abnormalities occurring during neoplasia.

Briefly these techniques utilize the ability of complementary single strands of DNA or RNA to reassociate (hybridize) to form a double-stranded molecular structure (Fig. 9.11). Labelled specific synthetic nucleotide sequences can act as probes for complementary segments of DNA or RNA present in a cell of interest. They will bind to their analogous DNA or RNA sequence in a preparation of nuclei acid from tissue or cells which have been separated and immobilized on synthetic filters (blotting). *In*

Schematic diagram of DNA hybridization procedure

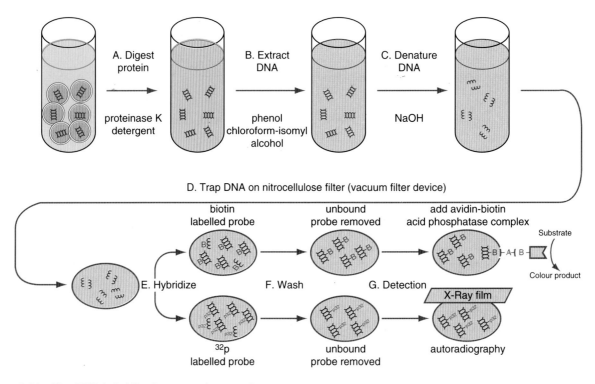

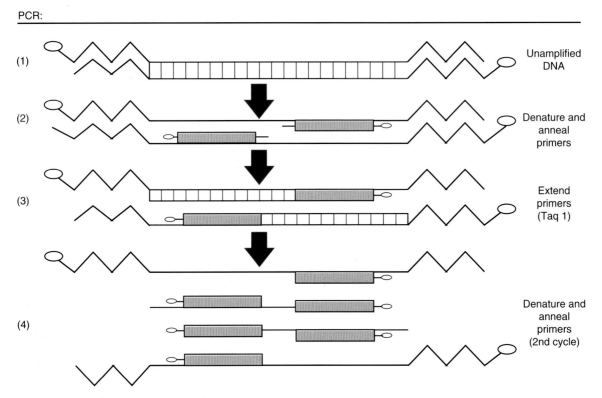

Figure 9.11 The DNA hybridization procedure can be used on tissue homogenized samples (blotting) or cell samples.

PCR:

Figure 9.12 The polymerase chain reaction.

situ hybridization uses similar concepts of binding between the labelled probe and a target sequence of DNA present in tissue or cells. The nucleic acid probe is identified through prior labelling with a radionucleotide or biotin. A radiolabelled probe can be identified using autoradiography and a biotin-related probe through immunocytochemical techniques. *In situ* hybridization thus allows qualitative as well as semiquantitative assessment of specific DNA or RNA changes in tumour cell populations as well as the site and frequency of occurrence of specific alterations [45].

The polymerase chain reaction (PCR) (Fig. 9.12) allows amplification of specific portions of DNA from small samples (theoretically a single cell). The product of the reaction can be assessed using conventional blotting technology or visualized using *in situ* hybridization as described earlier.

All of these molecular techniques can be applied to cytology samples but, perhaps, *in situ* hybridization, particularly in combination with PCR, has the most exciting potential as a cytology research tool [46]. This dual molecular method will amplify a single gene or part of a gene in a cell to a level where *in situ* hybridization can be used allowing visualization of the cells having very specific molecular genetic abnormalities.

The application of these methods to FNA samples could have a role in the diagnosis and classification of cancer, detection of early or preneoplastic changes and the identification of genetic changes which could influence response to the various forms of therapy available.

REFERENCES

1. Page, D. L. and Anderson, T. J. (1987) *Diagnostic Histopathology of the Breast*, Churchill Livingstone, Edinburgh.
2. Ellis, I. O., Galea, M. and Broughton, N. (1992) Pathological prognostic factors in breast cancer. II. Histological type. Relationship with survival in a large study with long-term follow-up. *Histopathol.* **20**, 479–89.
3. Mouriquand, J., Gozlan-Fior, M., Villemain, D. *et al.* (1986) Value of cytoprognostic classification in breast carcinomas. *J. Clin. Pathol.* **39**, 489–96.
4. Thomas, I. S., Mallon, E. A. and George, W. D. (1989) Semi-quantitative analyses of fine needle aspirates from benign and malignant breast lesions. *J. Clin. Pathol.* **42**, 28–34.
5. Cornelisse, C. J., de Koning, H. R. and Arentz, P. W. *et al.* (1981) Quantitative analysis of the nuclear area variation in benign and malignant breast cytology specimens. *Anal. Quant. Cytol.* **3**, 128–34.
6. Kuenen-Boumeester, V., Hop, W. C. J., Blonk, D. I. and Booon, M. E. (1984) Prognostic scoring using cytomorphometry and lymph node status of patients with breast carcinoma. *Eur. J. Cancer Clin. Oncol.* **20**, 337–45.
7. Zajdela, A., Riva, L. S. D. L. and Ghossein, N. A. (1979) The relation of prognosis to the nuclear diameter of breast cancer cells obtained by cytologic aspiration. *Acta Cytol.* **23**, 75–80.
8. Mossler, J. A., McCarty, K. S., Woodward, B. H. *et al.* (1982) Correlation of mean nuclear area with oestrogen receptor content in aspiration cytology of breast carcinoma. *Acta Cytol.* **26**, 417–21.
9. Wallgren, A., Silfversward, C. and Zajicek, J. (1976) Evaluation of needle aspirates and tissue sections as prognostic factors in mammary carcinoma. *Acta Cytol.* **20**, 313–8.
10. Hunt, C. M., Ellis, I. O., Elston, C. W. *et al.* (1990) Cytological grading of breast carcinoma – a feasible proposition? *Cytopathol.* **1**, 287–95.
11. Robinson, I. A., McKee, G., Nicholson, A. *et al.* (1994) Prognostic value of cytological grading of fine-needle aspirates from breast carcinoma. *Lancet*, **343**, 947–9.
12. Elston, C. W. and Ellis, I. O. (1991) Pathological prognostic factors in breast cancer. The value of histological grade in breast cancer: Experience from a large study with long-term follow up. *Histopathol.* **19**, 403–10.
13. Baak, J. P. A. and Oort, J. (1983) *A Manual of Morphometry in Diagnostic Pathology*, Springer, Berlin.
14. Brugal, G. (1984) Analysis of microscopic preparations, in *Methods and Achievements of Experimental Pathology*, (eds G. Jasmin and L. Proshek), Karger, Basel, pp. 1–33.
15. Hedley, D., Friedlander, M., Taylor, I. *et al.* (1983) Method for analysis of cellular DNA content of paraffin embedded pathological material using flow cytometry. *J. Histochem. Cytochem.* **31**, 1333.
16. Van Diest, P. J. and Baak, J. P. A. (1991) The morphometric prognostic index is the strongest prognosticator in premenopausal lymph node-negative and lymph node-positive breast cancer patients. *Hum. Pathol.* **22**, 326–30.
17. Wright, N. A. (1984) Cell proliferation in health and disease, in *Recent Advances in Histopathology*, (eds P. P. Anthony and R. N. M. MacSween), Chuchill Livingstone, Edinburgh, pp. 17–34.
18. Auer, G., Eriksson, E., Azavedo, E. *et al.* (1984) Prognostic significance of nuclear DNA content in mammary adenocarcinoma in humans. *Cancer Res.* **44**, 394–6.
19. Walker, R. and Camplejohn, R. (1986) DNA flow cytometry of human breast carcinomas and its relationship to transferrin and epidermal growth factor receptors. *J. Pathol.* **150**, 37–42.
20. Locker, A. P., Dilks, B., Gilmour, A. *et al.* (1990) Aspiration cytology diagnosis of breast lesions by nuclear DNA content. *Br. J. Surg.* **77**, A707.

21. Bocking, A., Adler, C. P., Common, H. H. *et al.* (1984) Algorithm for a DNA cytophotometric diagnosis and grading of malignancy. *Analyt. Quant. Cytometry,* **6,** 1–8.

22. Cornelisse, C. J. *et al.* (1985) DNA image cytometry on machine selected breast cancer cells and the comparison between flow cytometry and scanning cytophotometry. *Cytometry,* **6,** 471–7.

23. Hall, T. L. and Fu, Y. S. (1985) Applications of quantitative microscopy in tumour pathology. *Lab. Invest.* **53,** 5–21.

24. King, E. B., Chew, K. L., Duarte, L. *et al.* (1988) Image cytometric classification of pre-malignant disease in fine needle aspirates. *Cancer,* **62,** 114–24.

25. Baccas, S., Flowers, J. L., Press, M. E. *et al.* (1988) The evaluation of oestrogen receptor in primary breast carcinoma by computerised image analysis. *Am. J. Clin. Pathol.* **90,** 233–9.

26. Lovett, E. J., Schnitzer, B., Keren, D. F. *et al.* (1984) Application of flow cytometry to diagnostic pathology. *Lab. Invest* **50,** 115–40.

27. Giaretti, W. (1991) Ploidy and proliferation evaluated by flow cytometry. An overview of techniques and impact in oncology. *Tumori,* **77,** 403–19.

28. Remvikos, Y., Beuzebocp, P., Zajdela, A. *et al.* (1989) Correlation of proliferative activity of breast cancer with the response to cytotoxic chemotherapy. *J. Nat. Cancer Inst.* **81,** 1383–7.

29. Rew, D. A. and Wilson, G. D. (1991) Better understanding of the cell cycle could improve treatments for cancer. *Advances in Cell Kinetics. B.M.J.* **303,** 532–3.

30. Wilson, G. D., McNally, M. J., Dunphy, E. *et al.* (1985) The labelling index of human and mouse tumours assessed by bromodeoxyuridine staining *in vitro* and *in vivo* and flow cytometry. *J. Cytometry,* **6,** 641–7.

31. Wilson, G. D., McNally, N. J., Dische, S. *et al.* (1988) Measurement of cell kinetics in human tumours *in vivo* using bromodeoxyuridine incorporation and flow cytometry. *Br. J. Cancer,* **58,** 423–31.

32. Polak, J. M. and Van Noorden, S. (1986) *Immunocytochemistry: Modern Methods and Applications,* 2nd edn, Wright, Bristol.

33. Greene, G. L., Fitch, F. W. and Jensen, E. V. (1980) Monoclonal antibodies to estrophilin. *Proc. Natl. Acad. Sci. USA,* **77,** 157–61.

34. McCarty, K. S., Jr, Miller, L. S., Cox, E. B. *et al.* (1985) Oestrogen receptor analysis: correlation of biochemical and immunohistochemical methods using monoclonal antireceptor antibodies. *Arch. Pathol. Lab. Med.* **109,** 716–21.

35. Snead, D. R. J., Bell, J., Dixon, A. *et al.* (1993) Methodology of oestrogen receptor assessment on formalin fixed tissue. A comparison with traditional methods. *Histopathol.* **23,** 233–6.

36. Ryde, C. M., Smith, D., King, N. *et al.* (1992) Comparison of four immunochemical methods for the measurement of oestrogen receptor levels in breast cancer. *Cytopathology,* **3,** 155–60.

37. Robertson, J. F., Bates, K., Pearson, D. *et al.* (1992) Comparison of two oestrogen receptor assays in the prediction of the clinical course of patients with advanced breast cancer. *Br. J. Cancer* **65,** 727–30.

38. Locker, A. P., Birrell, K., Bell, J. A., *et al.* (1992) Ki67 immunoreactivity in breast carcinoma: relationships to prognostic variables and short term survival. *Eur. J. Surg. Oncol.* **18,** 224–9.

39. Gerdes, J. (1986) Growth fractions in breast cancers determined *in situ* with monoclonal antibody Ki-67. *J. Clin. Pathol.* **39,** 977.

40. Key, G., Becker, H. G., Baron, B. *et al.* (1992) Preparation and immunochemical characterization of new Ki-67 equivalent murine monoclonal antibodies (MIBI-3) generated against recombinant parts of the Ki-67 antigen.

41. Garcia, R. L., Coltrera, M. D. and Gown, A. M. (1989) Analysis of proliferative grade using anti-PCNA/cyclin monoclonal antibodies in fixed embedded tissues. *Am. J. Pathol.* **134,** 733–9.

42. Kuenen-Boumeester, V., Blonk, D. I. and Kwast, T. H. V. D. (1988) Immunocytochemical staining of proliferating cells in fine needle aspiration smears of primary and metastatic breast tumours. *Br. J. Cancer,* **57,** 509–11.

43. Morrow, C. S. and Cowan, K. H. (1988) Mechanisms and clinical significance of multidrug resistance. *Oncology,* **2,** 55–64.

44. Schneider, J., Bak, M., Efferth, T. *et al.* (1989) P-glycoprotein expression in treated and untreated human breast cancer. *Br. J. Cancer,* **60,** 815–8.

45. Goudie, R. B. (1989) DNA technology in histopathology, in *Recent Advances in Histopathology,* (eds P. Anthony and R. MacSween), Churchill Livingstone, Edinburgh.

46. Lonn, U., Lonn, S., Nylen, U. *et al.* (1991) Application of oncogenes in mammary carcinoma shown by fine needle biopsy. *Cancer,* **67,** 1396–400.

47. Heyderman, E., Steele, K. and Ormerod, M. (1979) A new antigen on the epithelial membrane: its immunoperoxidase localisation in normal and neoplastic tissues. *J. Clin. Pathol.* **32,** 35–9.

48. Hilkens, J., Buijs, F., Hilgers, J. *et al.* (1984) Monoclonal antibodies against human milk fat globule membranes detecting differentiation antigens of the mammary gland and its tumours. *Int. J. Cancer,* **34,** 197–206.

49. Price, M. R., Edwards, S., Owainati, A. *et al.* (1985) Multiple epitopes on a human breast carcinoma associated antigen. *Int. J. Cancer,* **36,** 567–74.

50. Gendler, S., Duhig, J. T.-P., Rothbard, J. and Burchell, J. (1988) A highly immunogenic region of human polymorphic epithelial mucin expressed by carcinomas is made up of tandem repeats. *J. Biol. Chem.* **263,** 12820–3.

51. Sainsbury, J., Farndon, J., Needham, G. *et al.* (1987) Epidermal growth factor receptor status as predictor of early recurrence of and death from breast cancer. *Lancet,* **2,** 1398–402.

52. Lewis, S., Locker, A., Todd, J. *et al.* (1990) Expression of epidermal growth factor receptor in breast carcinoma. *J. Clin. Pathol.* **43,** 385–98.

53. Sporn, M. and Roberts, A. B. (1985) Autocrine growth factors and cancer. *Nature*, **313**, 747–51.

54. Silberstein, G. B. and Daniel, C. W. (1987) Reversible inhibition of mammary gland growth by transforming growth factor β. *Science*, **237**, 291.

55. Venter, D. J., Kumar, S., Tuzi, N. and Gullick, W. J. (1987) Over-expression of the c-*erb*B-2 oncoprotein in human breast carcinomas: Immunohistochemical assessment correlated with gene amplification. *Lancet*, **ii**, 69–71.

56. Van-der-Vijver, M. J., Peterse, J. L., Mooi, W. J. *et al.* (1988) *Neu*-protein over expression in breast cancer: association with comedo-type ductal carcinoma *in situ* and limited prognostic value in stage II breast cancer. *N. Engl. J. Med.* **319**, 1239–45.

57. Lammie, G. A., Barnes, D. M., Millis, R. R. and Gullick, W. J. (1989) An immunohistochemical study of the presence of c-*erb*B-2 protein in Paget's disease of the nipple. *Histopathology*, **15**, 505–14.

58. Lovekin, C., Ellis, I. O., Locker, A. *et al.* (1991) c-*erb*B-2 oncoprotein expression in primary and advanced breast cancer. *Br. J. Cancer*, **63**, 439–43.

59. Slamon, D., Godolphin, W., Jones, L. *et al.* (1989) Studies of the HER-2/*neu* proto-oncogene in human breast and ovarian cancer. *Science*, **244**, 707–12.

60. Walker, R. A. and Wilkinson, N. (1988) p21 *ras* protein expression in benign and malignant human breast. *J.*

Pathol. **156**, 147–53.

61. Ohuchi, N., Thor, A., Page, D. L. *et al.* (1986) Expression of the 21000 molecular weight *ras* protein in a spectrum of benign and malignant human mammary tissues. *Cancer Res.* **46**, 2511–9.

62. Ghosh, A. K., Moore, M. and Harris, M. (1986) Immunohistochemical detection of *ras* oncogene p21 product in benign and malignant mammary tissue in man. *J. Clin. Pathol.* **39**, 428–34.

63. Locker, A., Dowle, C., Ellis, I. *et al.* (1989) C-*myc* oncogene product expression and prognosis in operable breast cancer. *Br. J. Cancer*, **60**, 669–72.

64. Meyer, J. and Friedman, L. (1983) Prediction of early course of breast carcinoma by thymidine labelling. *Cancer*, **51**, 1879–86.

65. Rochefort, H., Augereau, P. and Capony, F. (1988) The 52K cathepsin-D of breast cancer: Structure, regulation, function and clinical value, in *Breast Cancer: Cellular and Molecular Biology*, (eds M. E. Lippman and R. B. Dickson), Kluwer, Boston, pp. 207–22.

66. McGuire, W. L., Tandon, A. K., Allred, D. C. *et al.* (1990) How to use prognostic factors in axillary node-negative breast cancer patients. *J. Nat. Cancer Inst.* **82**(12), 1006–15.

67. Duffy, M. J., O'Grady, P., Devaney, D. *et al.* (1988) Tissue-type plasminogen activator, a new prognostic marker in breast cancer. *Cancer Res.* **48**, 1348–9.

Index

Numbers appearing in *italic* represent tables, those appearing in **bold** represent figures.

Aberrations of normal development
    and involution 17–19, 112
    see also Adenosis; Hyperplasia,
        atypical
Adenoid cystic carcinoma **5.12**, 98
Adenomas
    ductal 89–90, **5.3**
    lactating 16–17, **2.9**, **2.10**
    nipple 90, **6.20**, **6.21**
    pleomorphic 100, **5.16**
    tubular 88, **5.2**
    see also Adenomyoepithelioma;
        Fibroadenoma
Adenomyoepithelioma 100, **5.15**
Adenosis 17–19
    apocrine 91, **5.5**
    blunt duct 17
    microglandular 91–2
    sclerosing 17, **2.16**, **2.17**, 88
    nodular 99
Anti-hypertensive drugs 16
Antipsychotic drugs 16
Apocrine carcinoma 96–7, **5.10**
Aspiration cytodiagnosis
    accuracy 2, 3
        targets 124
    complications 4
    and histopathology 5–6, **4.21**
    historical aspects 2–3
    limitations 5, 139
    and management of breast disease
        3–4, 51, 139
    and metaplastic growth **4.9**
    needle biopsy comparison 4
    special training 3, 4
    techniques 6–8, **1.2**, **1.3**, **1.4**
Assessment clinic 134
Audit guidelines 124
Autoradiography 144

Bare nuclei, *see* Naked nuclei
Benign lesions
    atypical appearances **4.4**
    cytological indicators 15
Benign pairs, *see* Myoepithelial cells
Benign proliferative changes, *see*
        Aberrations of normal
        development and involution
Biopsy, needle
    aspiration cytodiagnosis
        comparison 4
    impalpable lesions 134

Biopty-gun 4
Breast development, normal 14
Breast pump 110
Breast structure, normal 14
    cytology **2.2**, **2.4**
    histology **2.3**

Cell cycle growth fraction **9.8**
    measurement
        flow cytometry 144–5
        immunocytochemistry 147
Centrifugation of samples 8
Classification
    of carcinomas 40, **3.2**
    of cytology, numerical 9–10, **9.1**,
        139, **9.2**
        proportions classified 51
    grading of carcinomas 39, **9.1**
    H-score system 146–7
Clinical categorization of aspirates 4
Collagenous spherulosis 92, **5.6**
    adenoid cystic carcinoma
        comparison 98
Colloid carcinoma 5
Comedo
    cytology **8.16**, **8.17**
    histology **8.15**
    image-guided aspiration 133
    see also *In situ* carcinoma
Complex sclerosing lesion 19–20, **8.12**,
        8.13, **8.14**
    image-guided aspiration 132–3
    see also Radial scar; Stellate lesion
Complications of aspiration
        cytodiagnosis 4
Connective tissue, stromal 14–15,
        2.14, **2.15**
Consistency of tumour 6
Cyst 22–3
    image-guided aspiration 130
    repeated aspiration **4.9**
    see also Cyst fluid; Epidermal cyst
Cyst fluid
    atypical, benign cytology **4.11**
    cytological examination 3, 22–3,
        2.30–6
    medullary carcinoma 46
Cytology clinic 6
Cytometry 140
    flow 143–5, **9.7**
    image 140–3, **9.2**

see also Cell cycle growth fraction;
    DNA quantitation

DNA quantitation 140, **9.3–6**, 144
Ductal hyperplasia 19, **2.18**, **2.19**
Duct ectasia 21, **2.24**, **2.26**, **6.9**, 113
Duct papilloma 113, **6.12–19**

Enzyme linked immunosorbent
        assays (ELISA) 146
Epidermal cyst 33, **2.66**, **2.67**
    see also Cyst
Epithelial cells
    and aberrations of normal
        development 17–19
    appearances in benign lesions 15
    breast cysts 23
    duct ectasia 21
    fibroadenoma 25, 27, **4.25**
        antiserum CALLA 27
    galactocoele 24
    gynaecomastia **5.4**
    in malignant lesions 36–8, **3.2**
    mastitis 28
    in normal tissue 14
    Paget's disease 117
    radial scars 20
    radiation changes 32
    suspicious of carcinoma **4.1**
Epithelial lesions, uncommon 89–98,
        5.1

False negative rate 122
    target value 124
False positive rate
    target value 124
Fat necrosis 30, **2.58**, **2.59**
Fibroadenoma
    changes in pregnancy 16
    cytodiagnosis 4, **2.40–6**, **3.6**
        cytology suspicious of carcinoma
            4.2, **4.6**, **4.12**
        misdiagnosis 5, 27–8, **4.19**, **4.25**
    histology **2.38**, **2.49**
    mammography 24–5, **2.39**, 130
    mucin **2.47**, 27–8
    oral contraceptives and 26
    phyllodes tumour comparison 99
    report style 9
Fibromatosis 101, **5.17**

Galactocoele 24, **2.37**, **6.7**

Granular cell tumour 101–2, **5.18**
Granulomatous mastitis 28–30
  cytology **2.55**, **2.56**
  histology **2.54**
  skin dimpling **2.57**
  see also Mastitis; Plasma cell mastitis
Gynaecomastia 90–1, **5.4**

Haemangiopericytoma 106
Hamartoma 103
Histopathology
  and cytopathology 5–6, **4.21**
Histoplasma 30
Historical aspects, aspiration
  cytodiagnosis 2–3
'Honeycombing' effect 15
H-score system 146–7
  see also Classification
Hyperplasia, atypical
  ductal 19, **2.18**, **2.19**, 94–5, **5.8**
  epithelial 19
  lobular 93–4, **5.7**

Image-guided aspiration 3, 127–9
  comedo 133
  complex sclerosing lesion 132–3
  diagnostic success, factors affecting
    129–30
  management options 134–5
  radial scar 132–3
  tubular carcinoma 130–2
Immunocytochemistry 144, **9.3**, 145–7
  angiosarcoma 105, **5.20**
  granular cell tumour **5.18**
  growth fraction measurement 147
  lymphoma cells 102, **5.19**
  resistance gene assay 147
Impalpable lesions
  biopsies of benign lesions 126–7
  categories 130–4
  diagnostic success, factors affecting
    129–30
  management 134–5
  physical examination 126
  radiological features 127
  range of diagnoses 130, **8.2**
Infiltrating carcinoma
  ductal
    cytology suspicious of carcinoma
      4.1, **4.3**, **4.5**, **4.24**
    medullary 3, 5, 45, **3.15**
    misinterpretation of cytology
      4.16, **4.19**
    mucoid 46, **3.16**
    NOS 40, 41–2, **3.7–11**
  lobular 43–4, **3.12**, **3.13**
    cytology suspicious of carcinoma
      4.8, **4.17**
    see also In situ carcinoma; Papillary
      carcinoma; Sarcoma
In situ carcinoma
  ductal **2.23**

cytology suspicious of carcinoma
  4.10
  misdiagnosis 105
  image-guided aspiration 133–4,
    8.15–17
  infiltrating carcinoma comparison
    44–5
  mammography **6.22**
  nipple smear 115–17, **6.23–6**
  oncogene positivity 36

Juvenile papillomatosis 88, **5.1**

Lactation 15–17
  cytology **2.5–8**
  nipple smear **6.3–6**
  see also Adenomas, lactating;
    Lactational carcinoma
Lactational carcinoma **3.3**
Langhans-type giant cells 28, **2.54**, 30
Lipoma 32, **2.62**, **2.63**
Lymph node, intramammary 32, **2.64**,
  2.65
Lymphoma 102, **5.19**

Malignant lesions
  classification 40, **3.2**
  criteria of malignancy 36–9, **3.1**, **3.2**,
    4.13, **4.22**
  cytological grading 39
Mammography
  calcification 127, **8.2**
  correlation with pathology **8.1**
  of cysts 22, **2.28**
  ductal carcinoma *in situ* **6.22**
  epidermal cysts 33
  fat necrosis 30
  fibroadenoma 24–5
  image-guidance 128–9, **8.6**, **8.7**
  limitations 4
  see also Image-guided aspiration;
    Stereotaxis
Mammotest 128
Management of breast disease
  cytological grading of cancers 139
  equivocal cases 51
  impalpable lesions 126–7, 134–5
  oestrogen receptor assay 147
  role of aspiration cytodiagnosis 3–4
Mastitis 28, **2.50**, **2.51**, 113, **6.11**
  see also Granulomatous mastitis;
    Plasma cell mastitis
Morphometry 140
Mucin
  fibroadenomas **2.47**, 27–8
  infiltrating carcinoma 42, **3.10**, **3.12**
Mucinous adenocarcinoma 5
Multidrug resistance gene product
  assay 147
Myoepithelial cells
  aberrations of normal development
    17–19

benign pairs 38, **3.5**, **4.6**
  fibroadenomas 27, **4.12**
  in normal tissue 14
  papillary carcinoma 46
  phyllodes tumour **4.23**
  radial scars 20
Myoepithelial lesions, uncommon **5.1**,
  99–101

Naked nuclei 15, **2.12**, **2.13**
  adenomyoepithelioma 100, **5.15**
  complex sclerosing lesion 133
  fibroadenoma 25, **2.43**, **2.46**
  infiltrating ductal carcinoma **4.16**
  pleomorphic adenoma 100, **5.16**
National Health Service Breast
  Screening Programme 88
  Forrest Report 126
  guidelines 9, 36, 51
  screening intervals 135
  statistical targets 124
Neuroendocrine carcinoma 98, **5.13**
Neuroendocrine differentiation 42,
  3.11
Neuroendocrine granules **4.13**, **4.15**
Nipple inversion 113
Nipple smear
  duct ectasia 21, **6.9**, **6.10**, 113
  duct papilloma 113, **6.12–19**
  galactocoele 112, **6.7**
  in situ carcinoma 115–17, **6.23–6**
  lactation 111–12, **6.3–6**
  mastitis 113, **6.11**
  nipple adenomas **6.20**, **6.21**
  normal **6.1**, **6.2**, 111
  Paget's disease 117–18, **6.27–9**
  papillary carcinoma **4.7**, **4.14**,
    113–15
  preparation 110
  Paget's disease 118
Nodular fasciitis 101, **5.17**
Nuclear appearance
  adenoid cystic carcinoma 98
  benign lesions 15
  cytology suspicious of carcinoma
    4.1, **4.7**
  granular cell tumour 102
  malignant lesions 36, *3.1*, **3.1**, **4.22**,
    4.24
  metaplastic cells **4.9**
  nodular sclerosing adenosis 99
  phyllodes tumour **4.23**
  see also Naked nuclei; Sentinel cells

Oestrogen receptor
  immunocytochemistry 146–7,
    9.9, **9.10**
Oncogenes 36
Oral contraceptives 26, 29, 110

Paget's disease of the nipple 117–18,
  6.27–9

Papillary carcinoma 46, **3.17**
  differentiation from papilloma **4.14**
  nipple smear **4.7**, 113–15
Papilloma, *see* Duct papilloma
Phenothiazines 106, 113
Phyllodes tumour **4.23**, 99, **5.14**
  stromal sarcoma comparison 106
Pituitary tumour 29
Plasma cell mastitis 21, **2.25**
  see also Duct ectasia;
      Granulomatous mastitis;
      Mastitis
Pneumothorax 4
Polymerase chain reaction (PCR) 149,
  9.12
Predictive value, aspiration
    cytodiagnosis 3, 122, *7.1*
  target value 124
Pregnancy, breast changes during
    15–16
Proliferation index, *see* Cell cycle
    growth fraction
Pseudosarcoma 9

Radial scar 19–20, **2.20–2**, 92, 132–3
  see also Complex sclerosing lesion;
      Stellate lesion
Radiation changes 31–2
  cytology **2.61**, **4.10**, **4.18**, **4.20**
  interpretation 5
  mammogram **2.60**
Recombinant DNA techniques 147–9,
  9.11

Reporting cytopathology 9–10
  see also Classification
Request forms 4

Sarcoidosis 30
Sarcoma 46–8, **3.18**
  angiosarcoma 103–5, **5.20**
  stromal 105–6, **5.21**
Sarcomatous metaplasia 9
Schwannoma 101
Sensitivity, aspiration cytodiagnosis
    3, 122, *7.1*
  and cytology clinics 6
  target value 124
Sentinel cells 15
Silicon granuloma 30
Small cell carcinoma **4.8**
  misdiagnosis 100
  see also Infiltrating carcinoma,
      lobular
Soft tissue lesions, uncommon *5.1*,
    101–6
Specificity, aspiration cytodiagnosis
    122, *7.1*
  and cytology clinics 6
  target value 124
Spiculate lesion, *see* Stellate lesion
Squamous carcinoma 97, **5.11**
Staining technique 6
Stellate lesion 19–20, *2.1*
  see also Complex sclerosing lesion;
      Radial scar
Stereotaxis 128–9, **8.6**, **8.7**

see also Ultrasonography
Stereotix 128–9
Stewart–Trieves syndrome 103
Subareolar abscess 28, **2.52**, **2.53**
Syringe holder 7, **1.2**

Target accuracy 124
Techniques of aspiration
    cytodiagnosis 6–8, **1.2–4**
Trauma, and fat necrosis 30
Trial of early detection of breast
    cancer 126
Triple diagnosis technique 3–4, 126
Tru-cut biopsy 4, 51, **4.17**
Tubular carcinoma 95–6, **5.9**, **8.9–11**
  image-guided aspiration 130–2
  microglandular adenosis
      comparison 92
Tumour seeding along needle tract 4

Ultrasonography
  of cysts 22, **2.29**, **8.3**
  fibroadenoma **8.4**
  image-guided aspiration 127–8, *8.3*
  results suspicious of malignancy **8.5**
  see also Image-guided aspiration

Vacuoles
  intracytoplasmic **4.2**, **4.7**, **4.16**, **4.21**,
      94
  intranuclear 36, **4.3**, **4.4**, **4.10**, **4.12**

Ziehl–Neilson stain 30

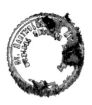